Clin-Alert® 2001

Clin-Alert® 2001

A Quick Reference to Adverse Clinical Events

Edited by

JOYCE GENERALI, MS, RPh, FASHP
Drug Information Center
University of Kansas

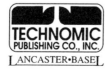

TECHNOMIC
PUBLISHING CO., INC.
LANCASTER•BASEL

Clin-Alert® 2001
aTECHNOMIC®publication

Technomic Publishing Company, Inc.
851 New Holland Avenue, Box 3535
Lancaster, Pennsylvania 17604 U.S.A.

Printed in the United States of America
10   9   8   7   6   5   4   3   2   1

Main entry under title:
    Clin-Alert® 2001: A Quick Reference to Adverse Clinical Events

A Technomic Publishing Company book
Bibliography: p.
Includes index p. 243

Library of Congress Catalog Card No. 00-112051
ISBN No. 1-58716-078-1

Contents

Acknowledgements

Many thanks and appreciation to Stephen Spangler, Bennett Rabiega, Michael B. Brown and the staff at Technomic Publishing Company for their hard work and efforts in making this book possible.

Recognition for continuing support to my family Steven, Jessica and Jonathan Whitfield and my parents Silvio and Vilma Generali.

Introduction

Keeping current with the safety profiles of drug therapy is essential in optimizing decisions regarding patient health care. However, with the addition of 25 to 30 new drugs to the United States market each year, this task becomes formidable. Although all drugs are tested for safety during premarketing trials, the full scope of the safety profile and drug interactions is not realized until the drug has been on the market for several years and used in a varied population in clinical scenarios that often involve polypharmacy. Thus, attention to potential side effects and drug interactions remains an important component of effective and rational drug therapy.

Changing safety profiles are not limited only to new drugs as new information is also published regarding new adverse reactions and/or drug interactions with older products. In addition, the popularity of alternative medicines and their use with conventional medicines has created a new need for information regarding drug interactions in this area.

The *Clin-Alert* newsletter is designed to collect, summarize and report newly published information regarding significant adverse drug events and drug interactions. In the last three years, the scope of the newsletter has expanded to include information on alternative medicines and herbal therapies, and to alert health care professionals regarding FDA notifications and public health advisories. This book is the second compilation of abstracts published in *Clin-Alert* and collates the reports presented in *Clin-Alert* for the last year. The abstracts are arranged by drug class and there are six indices for easy accessibility. This year a new index has been added which highlights adverse drug events with newly marketed agents (1997–2000).

Although most of the presented abstracts are summaries of published case reports, several abstracts also review data from drug interaction studies, prospective safety trials, case series or retrospective investigations. When the information is available a *Clin-Alert* abstract data regarding the suspected adverse event, the suspected drug (dose, duration of therapy and

ix

route of administration), concurrent therapy, onset of action of the event, management or treatment of the side effect, relevant laboratory or physical examination data, dechallenge and rechallenge information, and clinical outcome. In addition, the author's conclusion and suggested mechanism of actions are provided. Full reference citations with reprint address and author's e-mail address (if available) are provided for ease of access to further information if needed. In addition, web page citations are included for easy access to information regarding FDA notifications or online journal access via the Internet.

It should be noted that these abstracts summarize reported information and that definitive causality is difficult to assess from case report data. Patient care decisions should never be based on abstract data alone and the reader is encouraged to access the original publication when needed. Abstracts are a useful tool in keeping current with the published literature and in identifying which articles may be of particular interest for the reader.

Adverse reactions and drug interactions are a dynamic part of a drug therapy. I am hopeful that this book will be a useful addition to the reader's library.

Joyce Generali, MS, RPh, FASHP
Director, Drug Information Center
University of Kansas Medical Center

ALTERNATIVE MEDICINES
ALTERNATIVE MEDICINES
ALTERNATIVE MEDICINES
ALTERNATIVE MEDICINES
ALTERNATIVE MEDICINES
ALTERNATIVE MEDICINES

Drug	Interacting Drug	ADR	Page Number
Androstenedione		Priapism	3
Aristolochic Acid		Nephrotoxicity	3
Averrhoa Carambola		Death in uremia^	4
Chromium picolinate		Exanthematous pustulosis*	4
Creatine	Ma Huang	Ischemic stroke*	8
Ecabalium elaterium		Uvular angioedema	5
Henna		Cutaneous reactions	6
Henna		Hemolysis	5
Herbal vitamins		Lead intoxication	6
Kampo		Epithelial keratopathy*	7
Laminaria tents		Bacteremia	7
Ma Huang	Creatine	Ischemic stroke*	8
St. John's wort	Cyclosporine	Cyclosporine concentrations decreased	10, 11
St. John's wort	Digoxin	Digoxin levels decreased	11
St. John's wort	Indinavir	Indinavir concentrations decreased	9

* = first report
^ = death
(+) = legal action

Alternative Medicines

ANDROSTENEDIONE
Priapism

A 30-year-old man developed priapism after starting androstenedione (1 pill daily) one week earlier. He did not seek medical attention until the episode had lasted for 30 hrs. There were no concurrent medications but a medication history revealed a previous episode one year earlier (duration: two to three hours) while taking the same supplement. Therapy included corpora cavernosa aspiration, normal saline irrigation and intracavernous injection with phenylephrine. Alternate etiologies were excluded. The authors suggested that androstenedione, a precursor of testosterone, increased serum testosterone levels in this patient, and possibly resulted in a hypersensitivity to erectile blood flow and an increased risk of priapism.

Kachi PN & Henderson SO (Henderson SO, Dept Emerg Med, LAC+USC Med Center, Unit #1, Room 1011, 1200 N Stone St, Los Angeles, CA 90033; e-mail: sohender@hsc.usc.edu) Priapism after androstenedione intake for athletic performance enhancement. Ann Emerg Med 35(4):391–393 (Apr) 2000

ARISTOLOCHIC ACID
Nephrotoxicity, FDA Advisory

On June 1, 2000, the FDA notified health professionals regarding potential nephrotoxicity associated with botanical products containing aristolochic acid. Although the FDA has not received similar adverse events, in July 1999, two new cases were reported in England regarding nephropathy associated with the use of Chinese botanical preparations containing this product. (See Clin Alert: 1999, 37:207) End stage renal disease cases were also reported in Belgium after ingestion of diet pills containing the same botanical. The FDA encouraged health care professionals to report adverse events, which occur during therapy with alternative medicines or botanical products. A complete list of products containing aristolochic acid can be found at http://vm.cfsan.fda.gov/~dms/ds-bot2.html

Letter to health care professionals on FDA concern about botanical products including dietary supplements containing aristolochic acid. (Jun 1) 2000 http://vm.cfsan.fda.gov/~dms/ds-bot2. html

AVERRHOA CARAMBOLA (STAR FRUIT)
Death in Uremic Patients

Over a nine year period, 20 uremic patients (mean age: 53.8 yrs) were hospitalized with acute neurological symptoms after ingesting star fruit or juice. Symptoms included limb numbness (15), persistent hiccups (12), altered consciousness (10), decreased muscle strength (7), dyspnea (5) and skin paresthesias (1). Patients were receiving regular hemodialysis (15), peritoneal dialysis (4) or in chronic renal failure without dialysis (1). Of the eight patients who died after ingestion (mean age: 56.6 yrs), all had eaten one to two fresh fruits with subsequent symptom onset between 2.5 and 14 hours. Symptom onset was shorter in patients who died than in those who had survived (mean: 4.6 vs 8.8 hrs). Hyperkalemia was evident in only four patients. Otherwise, serum calcium and potassium were within normal ranges. Treatment included emergent or routine dialysis in 10 patients each.

The authors cautioned that renal failure patients undergoing dialysis might develop neurological complications that could potentially be fatal after ingesting star fruit. Although star fruit has a high potassium content, hyperkalemia occurred in only four patients.

Chang JM et al (Lai YH, Div Nephrology, Dept Med, Kaoshiung Med Univ, 100 Shih-Chuan 1st Rd, Kaoshiung 807, Taiwan; e-mail:jemich@cc.kmc.edu.tw) Fatal outcome after ingestion of star fruit (averrhoa carambola) in uremic patients. Am J Kidney Diseases 35(2):189–293 (Feb) 2000

CHROMIUM PICOLINATE
Exanthematous Pustulosis (First Report*)

A 32-year-old patient developed a generalized erythematous pustular rash with low-grade fever approximately four days after starting chromium picolinate (1 gram daily) for nutritional supplementation. No other prescription or nonprescription medications were taken. The eruption consisted of several nonfollicular pustules on the trunk and extremities. Laboratory tests did not indicate an infection as evidenced by normal white blood cell counts. Skin punch biopsy revealed that the pustules contained neutrophils and eosinophils without infectious origins. Treatment included an oral prednisone tapering regimen (60 mg daily) over 15 days and oral dicloxacillin (1 gm daily) for one week. Chromium picolinate was also discontinued at this time. The eruption resolved within one week after treatment. Patch testing with chromium picolinate in various concentrations was negative. Rechallenge was not attempted due to the severity of the initial reaction. Despite negative patch testing, the authors concluded that this patient's cutaneous reaction was temporally related to chromium picolinate administration.

Young PC et al (Dermatol Service, Walter Reed Army Med Center, Washington, District of Columbia) Acute generalized exanthematous pustulosis induced by chromium picolinate. J Am Acad Dermatol 41:820–823 (Nov) 1999

ECBALIUM ELATERIUM
Uvular Angioedema

A 54-year-old woman developed dyspnea and sore throat approximately five hours after aspirating an intranasal alternative medicine (Ecbalium elaterium) for sinusitis. Upon hospitalization she was hypertensive (140/100 mmHg) and tachycardic (100 bpm) with an increased respiratory rate (34/min). In addition, the patient had severe uvular angioedema. Other medications included amoxicillin/clavulanate (1 gram twice daily) and naproxen sodium (550 mg twice daily). Gradual improvement occurred over 1.5 hours after supportive therapy was initiated, including intravenous epinephrine (0.3 mg) and prednisolone (80 mg). Further recovery was uneventful and the patient was discharged.

The authors noted that ecbalium elaterium is more commonly called "squirting cucumber" and often used as a folk medicine for sinusitis. They concluded that this patient's experience probably was a result of a local allergic reaction to a small amount of aspirated product. They also cautioned that patients who develop dyspnea after inhalation of "squirting cucumber" should seek immediate medical attention.

Eray O et al (Dept Emerg Med, Dokuz Eylul Univ, Balcova, 35340 Izmir, Turkey) Severe uvular angioedema caused by intranasal administration of ecbalium elaterium. Vet Human Toxicol 41(6):376–378 (Dec) 1999

HENNA
Acute Hemolysis

An 11-year-old patient was hospitalized for paleness, weakness and red colored urine, which occurred within 24 hours after total body henna application. A physical examination upon admission revealed reddish brown hued psoriatic lesions over the entire body surface area, predominantly on the extensor side of the extremities. Abnormal laboratory values included hemoglobin (4.5 gm/dL), hematocrit (13%), white blood cell count

(6700/mm^3), platelet count (342,000/mm^3), BUN (90 mg/dL), aspartate aminotransferase (420 IU/L), alanine aminotransferase (104 IU/L), indirect bilirubin (5.2 mg/dL), and creatine kinase (254 IU/dL). Treatment with transfusion and supportive care resulted in eventual recovery. The authors concluded that lawsone, a primary ingredient in henna, was substantially absorbed after topical application and was responsible for hemolysis in G6PD deficient red blood cells.

Soker M et al. (Dept Ped, Dicle Univ Faculty Med, Diyarbakir, Turkey; e-mail:sokerm @hotmail.com) Henna induced acute hemolysis in a G6PD deficient patient: A case report. Int Pediatrics 15(2):114–116 (Jul) 2000

HENNA
Cutaneous Reactions

In the past decade, henna induced cutaneous reactions were observed in 14 adult women (ages: 18 to 52 years) seeking medical attention at a Taiwan hospital. Six patients were successfully treated with potent topical corticosteroids and declined further study. Of the remaining eight patients who were patch tested for allergic responses, two exhibited a positive response to plain henna and six had a positive response to common additives in henna products.

The authors concluded that these findings support data that true henna allergy is a rare event. The allergens that are usually responsible for cutaneous reactions after henna application are most likely scented oils and additives, such as p-phenylenediamine.

Lestringant GG et al (Dept Dermatol, Taiwan Univ Hosp, PO Box 15258, Al Ain, United Arab Emirates; e-mail:hhlest@emirates.net.ae) Cutaneous reactions to henna and associated additives. Br J Dermatol 141:573–609 (Sep) 1999 (letter)

HERBAL VITAMINS
Lead Intoxication

A 5-year-old patient with encephalopathy, seizures and developmental delay as a result of neonatal asphyxia was noted to have an elevated lead concentration (86 mcg/dL) during an evaluation for persistent anemia. A repeated medication history revealed that the mother had been administering a Tibetan herbal vitamin three times daily for the last four years. A physical examination after hospitalization revealed a nonverbal child who was alert, but was unable to ambulate. Skeletal and abdominal x-rays did not reveal lead lines or particles, respectively. Chelation therapy with EDTA and BAL decreased the lead levels to 25.6 mcg/dL. Urinary lead excretion was 5578 mcg/24 hour urine. Analysis of the vitamin tablets revealed that the product contained lead, arsenic, cadmium, and mercury.

Lead ingestion over a four-year period was estimated at 63 grams. Repeat analysis of the 24 hour urine sample revealed the additional presence of mercury (28.64 mcg/24 hr urine) but arsenic was undetectable. Serum concentrations of mercury were undetectable and arsenic levels were 0.2 mcg/dL. Over the next four year period six additional chelation treatments were administered with succimer, resulting in the most recent lead level of 24.5 mcg/dL.

The authors concluded that this patient's lead intoxication was due to the ingestion of an herbal medicine as testing at the home site was negative for other lead sources.

Moore C & Adler R (Div Gen Pediatrics, Children's Hosp Los Angeles, Los Angeles, CA 90027) Herbal vitamins: Lead toxicity and developmental delay. Pediatrics 106(3): 600–602 (Sep) 2000

KAMPO (CHINESE HERBAL)
Epithelial Keratopathy (First Report*)

A 30-year-old patient developed bilateral photophobia during chronic therapy with an oral oriental herbal medicine, used to treat constipation, for five years. Composition of the herbal medicine included extracts from the scutellaria root, glycyrrhiza root, patycodon root, gypsum, atractylodes rhizome, rhubarb rhizome, schizopepeta spike, gardenia fruit, peony root, cridium rhizome, Japanese angelica root, mentha herb, saposhnikovia root, ephedra herb, forsythia fruit, ginger rhizome, talc, and anhydrous mirabilitum. A slit lamp examination revealed dust like opacities in the epithelial layers of both corneas and brown colored precipitates. No other concurrent medications were taken at this time. Two years prior to this event, similar ocular symptoms occurred, but reversed after withdrawal of the herbal medicine. At withdrawal of the drug this time, the corneal opacities decreased within three months and reversed completely within one year. No recurrences have been noted within four years of follow-up.

The authors concluded that this is the first case report of oriental herbal medicine induced keratopathy.

Akatsu T et al (Dept Ophthalmol, Juntendo Univ, Sch Med) Oriental herbal medicine induced epithelial keratopathy. Br J Ophthalmol 84:934 (Sep) 2000 (letter)

LAMINARIA TENTS
Bacteremia

A 26-year-old woman developed fever and shaking chills within 24 hours after laminaria tents were placed intravaginally in preparation for a planned abortion. Symptoms reversed with acetaminophen (no dosage provided) and the elective procedure was performed under sterile conditions. The fever and chills recurred post-procedure requiring hospitalization for suspected infection. Upon admission, the patient had a fever of 104 degrees Fahrenheit and was hypotensive (100/80 mmHg). Although a physical examination was normal, the white blood cell count was 1,400/mL with 79% neutrophils. Urine cultures were negative, but blood cultures revealed K. pneumoniae and group B streptococcus. Ceftriaxone and clindamycin therapy was switched to intravenous ampicillin/sulbactam. Although a superficial venous thrombosis was noted at the catheter placement site, recovery was uneventful and the patient was discharged on oral levofloxacin.

The authors concluded that although the laminaria tents were sterile, their placement inadvertently transferred flora from the vaginal tract into the uterine cavity, thus causing an infection.

Acharya PS & Gluckman SJ (Div of Infectious Dis & Dept Internal Med, Hosp of Univ Pennslyvania, Phildelphia, PA) Bacteremia following placement of intracervical laminaria tents. Clin Infectious Diseases 29:695–696 (Sep) 1999 (letter)

MA HUANG AND CREATINE
Ischemic Stroke (First Report*)

A 33-year-old body builder developed aphasia and right sided face and arm weakness approximately six weeks after starting athletic performance enhancers, Ma Huang and creatine products. He was taking no other medications at the time. Two capsules of the Ma Huang product contained ephedra alkaloids (20 mg), caffeine (200 mg), L-carnitine (100 mg), and chromium (200 mcg). One scoop of the powdered product contained creatine monohydrate (6000 mg), taurine (100 mg), inosine (100 mg), and co-enzyme Q10 (5 mg). Prior to his stroke he ingested 40 to 60 mg ephedra alkaloids and 400 to 600 mg of caffeine daily. A CT scan of the brain revealed an extensive left middle cerebral artery infarct. However, normal results were obtained via cerebral angiography, CSF examination, cardiac examinations, and cervical ultrasound. Creatinine was high but within normal ranges (102 umol/L).

The authors concluded that the combination of high dose ephedra and creatine were most likely responsible for ischemic stroke in this patient. They also suggested that caffeine may have enhanced the cardiovascular effects of ephedrine. According to the authors this is the first case report of cerebral infarct associated with high doses of these products. They also cautioned clinicians to alert the sports community of the potential risks of energy supplements.

Vahedi K et al (Serv Neurol, Hosp Lariboisiere, 2 Rue A Pare, 75010, Paris, France; e-mail:vahedi@ccr.jussieu.fr) Ischaemic stroke in a sportsman who consumed Ma Huang extract and creatine monohydrate for body building. J Neuro Neurosurg Psychiatry 68:112–113 (Jan) 2000

ST. JOHN'S WORT AND INDINAVIR
Interaction: Decreased Indinavir Concentrations, FDA Advisory

On February 10th, 2000 the FDA published a public health advisory regarding a recent NIH study which demonstrated a significant drug interaction between St. John's wort (hypericum perforatum) and indinavir. Concurrent administration resulted in decreased indinavir concentrations possibly related to cytochrome P450 isoenzyme induction. The FDA recommended that St. John's wort should not be used concurrently with any of the currently marketed protease inhibitors or nonnucleoside transcriptase inhibitor antiretrovirals as suboptimal plasma concentrations may reduce virologic response and promote resistance. The FDA is working with manufacturers of the antiretrovirals to revise product labeling to include these new recommendations.

FDA Public Health Advisory. Risk of drug interactions with St. John's wort and indinavir and other drugs. (Feb 10) 2000. http://www.fda. gov/cder/drug/advisory/stjwort.htm

ST. JOHN'S WORT AND INDINAVIR
Interaction: Decreased Indinavir Concentrations

In an open label study, eight healthy male volunteers (age range: 29 to 50 yrs) received indinavir alone (800 mg) every eight hours for four doses. After monotherapy plasma concentrations were obtained, St. John's wort (300 mg three times daily) was administered with meals for 14 days. Four doses of indinavir (800 mg every eight hours on an empty stomach) therapy were administered during the last two days of St. John's wort therapy. Although time to maximum indinavir concentrations were unchanged with or without St. John's wort administration (1.1 hrs), the mean AUC at eight hours was decreased by 57% when administered with the herbal product (30.8 mcg.hr/mL vs 12.3 mcg.hr/mL). Concurrent administration also resulted in reduced indinavir concentrations at eight hours by a range of 49% to 99%. Mean maximum concentrations were also reduced (12.3 mcg/mL to 8.9 mcg/mL).

The authors concluded that indinavir plasma concentrations are significantly reduced by concurrent St. John's wort therapy most likely via CYP3A4 isoenzyme induction. Because other antiretrovirals are also metabolized by the same isoenzyme system, they recommended that these combinations be avoided until further information is available.

Piscitelli SC et al (Dept Pharmacy, Warren G Magnuson Clin Center & Lab of Immunoregulation, NIH, Bethesda, MD 20892; e-mail:spisc@nih.gov) Indinavir concentrations and St. John's wort. Lancet 355:547 (Feb 12) 2000 (letter)

ST. JOHN'S WORT AND CYCLOSPORINE
Interaction: Heart Transplant Rejection

Two cases of failed heart transplants are presented in patients who had reduced cyclosporine levels while taking the alternative medicine, St. John's Wort.

Patient #1: A 61-year-old patient previously stabilized after a heart transplant 11 months earlier was hospitalized with fatigue three weeks after starting St. John's wort (300 mg three times daily) for depression. Other chronic medications included cyclosporine (125 mg twice daily), azathioprine (100 mg daily), and corticosteroids (7.5 mg daily). Prior to St. John's wort therapy cyclosporine levels had been consistently within therapeutic range but upon admission they were decreased (95 mcg/L). Endomyocardial biopsy revealed acute cellular transplant rejection. Despite stopping St. John's wort therapy, increasing cyclosporine dosages (150 mg twice daily) and intravenous steroid dosing (1 gram/day), rejection status was unchanged. However, permanent rejection was avoided by treatment substitution with mycophenolate mofetil (1 gram twice daily) and short term intravenous anti-thymocyte globulin (1250 mg daily for 10 days). Cyclosporine levels returned to baseline levels after St. John's wort therapy was stopped.

Patient #2: A 63-year-old patient previously stabilized after a heart transplant 20 months earlier was hospitalized for elective endomyocardial biopsy three weeks after starting St. John's wort (300 mg three times daily) for anxiety and depression. Other chronic medications included cyclosporine (125 mg twice daily), azathioprine (125 mg daily), and corticosteroids (7.5 mg daily). Prior to St. John's wort therapy cyclosporine levels had been consistently within therapeutic range but upon admission they were decreased (87 mcg/L). Endomyocardial biopsy revealed acute cellular transplant rejection. Cyclosporine levels returned to therapeutic range after St. John's wort therapy was stopped and no further rejection episodes occurred during follow-up.

The authors concluded that in both patients, St. John's wort therapy was associated with a reduction in cyclosporine plasma concentrations and subsequent transplant rejection episodes. After stopping St. John's wort treatment, cyclosporine concentrations returned to therapeutic range, and rejection episodes were reversed. The authors suggested that cyclosporine levels were decreased via cytochrome P450 induction via St. John's wort. As this is an interaction with serious consequences clinicians are encouraged to avoid this combination.

Ruschitzka F et al (Division of Cardiology, Dept Internal Med, Univ Hosp, C4-8091 Zurich, Switzerland) Acute heart transplant rejection due to Saint John's wort. Lancet 355:548 (Feb 12) 2000 (letter)

ST. JOHN'S WORT AND CYCLOSPORINE
Drug Interaction: Decreased Cyclosporine Concentrations, Transplant Rejection

A 29-year-old renal/pancreatic transplant patient, previously stabilized on cyclosporine with whole blood concentrations ranging from 250 to 300 ng/mL, developed decreased levels after self medicating with St. John's wort for mood elevation. Maintenance cyclosporine therapy was 100 mg twice daily. Other medications, which were unchanged during this time, included prednisone (10 mg daily) for immunosuppression and oral clonidine (0.2 mg twice daily) for hypertension. The patient denied other new prescription drug use but did not identify herbal product use. Within 30 days after starting St. John's wort cyclosporine trough concentrations decreased to 155 ng/mL and continued to drop when repeat measurements were performed three weeks later (97 ng/mL). Serum amylase increases (314 U/L) with abdominal pain suggested acute transplant rejection, which was verified by a renal biopsy. Treatment included antithymocyte globulin (20 mg/kg/day for two weeks) and cyclosporine dosage increases (175 mg twice daily). St. John's wort use, discovered at this time, was discontinued. After two weeks at increased dosages trough concentrations increased to 510 ng/mL and eventually stabilized between 200 to 350 ng/mL at previous doses. Serum amylase concentrations did not return to baseline and the patient experienced chronic organ rejection, requiring dialysis.

The authors suggested that acute transplantation rejection occurred in this patient as a result of subtherapeutic cyclosporine levels via CYP3A4 isoenzyme induction and/or P-glycoprotein pump activity, both induced by St. John's wort. They recommended that patient medication interviews should include specific inquiries about alternative medicine and herbal product use.

Barone GW et al (Dept Surgery, Slot 520-4, Univ Arkansas Med Sciences, 4301 W. Markham St, Little Rock, AR 72205; e-mail:baronegary@exchange.uams.edu) Drug interaction between St. John's wort and cyclosporine. Ann Pharmacother 34:1013–1016 (Sep) 2000

ST JOHN'S WORT AND DIGOXIN
Interaction: Decreased Digoxin Levels

In a single blinded, placebo controlled parallel study, 25 healthy volunteers (mean age: 26 yrs) received an oral loading dose of digoxin (0.25 mg twice daily) for two days followed by once daily dosing for an additional 13 days. Steady state serum concentrations were collected on day five and patients were then allocated to receive either placebo or St. John's wort three times daily for 10 days. Each enteric-coated active treatment tablet contained hypericin (92 mcg), pseudo hypericin (262 mcg) and hyperforin (18.37 mcg). After combination therapy for 10 days, mean half-life (42.8 vs 39.5 hrs) and median time to maximum concentrations (1 hr) were not different when compared to digoxin therapy alone. However, AUC values were decreased by 25 (17.2 vs 12.9 mcg/h/L), C_{max} was decreased by 26 (1.9 vs 1.4 mcg/L) and trough concentrations were decreased by 19 (0.58 vs 0.47 mcg/L). In contrast, the AUC values of hypericin and pseudo hypericin were unchanged when administered alone or with digoxin.

The authors concluded that St. John's wort might reduce the efficacy of digoxin via lowered AUC levels and trough concentrations. They theorized that digoxin kinetics are altered by hypericin extract induced P-glycoprotein activity.

Johne A et al (I Roots, Instit of Clin Pharmacol, Charite, Humboldt Univ of Berlin, Schumannstrasse 20/21, D-10098 Berlin, Germany) Pharmacokinetic in-teraction of digoxin with an herbal extract from St. John's wort (hypericum perforatum). Clin Pharmacol & Ther 66:338–345 (Oct) 1999

ANTIINFECTIVES

ANTIINFECTIVES

ANTIINFECTIVES

ANTIINFECTIVES

ANTIINFECTIVES

ANTIINFECTIVES

Drug	Interacting Drug	ADR	Page Number
General			
Antibiotics		Rash in pediatric patients	17
Aminoglycoside			
Gentamicin		Neurotoxicity, ototoxicity (+)	18
Antifungals			
Fluconazole		QT prolongation	19
Fluconazole		Fixed drug eruption	18
Itraconazole	Clarithromycin	Clarithromycin concentrations increased	35
Ketoconazole	Amprenavir	Increased concentrations	23
Miconazole (vaginal)	Warfarin	INR increased*	19
Antivirals			
Antiretroviral		Lipodystrophy, curly hair	20
Antiretroviral	Methylprednisolone	Immunosuppression (+)	21
Abacavir		Hypersensitivity reactions^	21
Amantadine		CNS ADRs	22
Amprenavir		Propylene glycol toxicity (potential)	23
Amprenavir	Ketoconazole	Increased concentrations	23
Indinavir	St. John's wort	Indinavir concentrations decreased	25
Indinavir		Crystalluria	24
Protease inhibitors		Hyperglycemia	27
Protease inhibitors		Hyperprolactinemia	26
Ritonavir	Meperidine	Meperidine concentrations increased	28
Ritonavir	Fentanyl	Fentanyl clearance decreased	27
Ritonavir		Hepatoxicity in hepatitis C or B	29

Drug	Interacting Drug	ADR	Page Number
Ritonavir	Methadone	Methadone effect decreased	28
Saquinavir		Hypoglycemia	29
Valacyclovir		Thrombotic thrombocytopenic purpura	30
Zanamivir		Respiratory distress	31
Cephalosporins			
Cefazolin		Fever	31
Cefdinir		Red stools	32
Cefotetan		Hemolysis	32
Ceftazidime	Vancomycin	Ocular precipitation (intravitreal)	33
Cefuroxime		Lymphomatoid hypersensitivity	34
Macrolides			
Clarithromycin	Omeprazole	Omeprazole concentrations increased	34
Clarithromycin	Itraconazole	Clarithromycin concentrations increased	35
Erythomycin		Pyloric stenosis (infantile)	36
Miscellaneous			
Bacitracin		Anaphylaxis	37
Quinupristin Dalfopristin		Hyponatremia	37
Vancomycin	Ceftazidime	Ocular precipitation (intravitreal)	33
Quinolones			
Alatrovafloxacin		Thrombocytopenia*	38
Ciprofloxacin	Warfarin	Hypothrombinemia, bleeding	41
Ciprofloxacin		Allergy	39
Ciprofloxacin		Tendon rupture	40
Ciprofloxacin		Bullous pemphigoid*	39
Ciprofloxacin	Glyburide	Hypoglycemia (resistant)	40
Levofloxacin		QT prolongation*	42
Trovafloxacin		Neurotoxicity	42
Trovafloxacin		Eosinophilic hepatitis	43
Trovafloxacin		Demylinating polyneuropathy*	43
Sulfonamides			
Trimethoprim Sulfamethoxazole		Stevens Johnson syndrome^ (+)	44
Trimethoprim Sulfamethoxazole		Hypokalemia in renal transplant patients	44

Drug	Interacting Drug	ADR	Page Number
Tetracyclines Minocycline Minocycline Tetracycline		Chest pain Hyperpigmentation (tongue) Pseudotumor cerebri (+)	46 46, 47 47
* = first report ^ = death (+) = legal action			

Antiinfectives

GENERAL
ANTIBIOTICS
Rash in Pediatric Patients

The frequency and severity of antibiotic rashes was investigated in a retrospective review of 5923 medical records of pediatric patients cared for in a community practice setting over a five month period. Approximately one-third (32%) of the patients did not receive antibiotics during this time period. However, antibiotic related reactions were documented in 8.6% (509) of the patients with 37 of these reactions classified as mild (e.g., gastrointestinal upset). The remaining 472 reactions were rash related. Of these reactions, there were no significant differences between the total number of boys and girls (53.8% vs 47.2%) who developed rashes, but there was a higher incidence observed in boys younger than three years of age, and in girls older than nine years. The highest incidence of reported rashes occurred in children who received cefaclor (12.3%), penicillins (7.4%), sulfonamides (8.5%), and other cephalosporins (2.6%). Urticarial type rashes (e.g., welts, hives, etc) were the most common, accounting for 45.9% (208) of the describable rashes. Thirty-one cases of serum sickness-like reactions were also observed in this patient population and were most frequently associated with cefaclor (1.9%), but also occurred in patients receiving penicillins (0.35%) and sulfonamides (0.36%). During the study period, no cases of severe rash related reactions (e.g., Stevens-Johnson syndrome, toxic epidermal necrolysis) occurred. In addition, there were no deaths or hospitalizations related to antibiotic induced rashes.

The authors concluded that antibiotic related rashes occurred in approximately 7% of the pediatric patients treated in a private pediatric practice. A significantly higher incidence of rash was associated with the use of cefaclor.

Ibia EO et al. (Dept Infectious Dis, Children's Nat Med Center, Washington DC) Antibiotic rashes in children. A survey in a private practice setting. Arch Dermatol 136:849–854 (Jul) 2000

AMINOGLYCOSIDES
GENTAMICIN
Excessive Dosage: Neurotoxicity and Ototoxicity, Legal Action

A three-week-old inpatient received intravenous ampicillin (160 mg) and gentamicin (8.5 mg) every 12 hours in the hospital and was discharged to home infusion therapy with continued therapy for two days. Unfortunately, the prescription was inadvertently changed to seven days and this amount was administered via a home infusion company over the next seven days. The patient developed vestibular dysfunction and severe deafness and may be prone to nephrotoxicity. The plaintiff alleged negligence on the part of the hospital and home infusion company for excessive dosage and inadequate monitoring, respectively. The case was settled for a total expected payment of $5,050,855 until the age of 50 yrs.

Doe vs Doe Excessive dosage of gentamicin through in-home IV antibiotic therapy—neurotoxic effect—vestibular dysfunction, permanent hearing loss—Utah Settlement for $5,050,855. Hosp Med Malpractice Verdicts, Settlements & Experts 16(3):25 (Mar) 2000

ANTIFUNGALS
FLUCONAZOLE
Fixed Drug Eruption

A 36-year-old patient received 18 doses of fluconazole over a 44-month period for recurrent candidal vulvovaginitis. Approximately three years after the initial fluconazole exposure the patient developed a red macule on the left thigh and fourth finger after fluconazole dosing. Although the macules resolved spontaneously within a few days, violet pigmentation persisted on the thigh. Painful blistering also occurred during two subsequent fluconazole regimens. One year later, erythematous patches developed at the same thigh and finger sites, approximately 12 hours post fluconazole dosing. Local testing with topical fluconazole (10%) product was applied on the affected areas of the thigh, finger and normal skin of the back. Within 24 hours, a red patch developed on the thigh only. Histological examination revealed a lichenoid infiltration consistent with a fixed drug eruption.

The authors concluded that fluconazole was responsible for a fixed drug eruption in this patient. Mechanism of action is unknown but may be related to a delayed allergic reaction.

Heikkila H et al (Dept Dermatol & Venerol, Helsinki Univ Central Hosp, Meilahdentie 2, 00250 Helsinki 25, Finland; email:hannele.heikkila@pp.inet.fi) Fixed drug eruption due to fluconazole. J Am Acad Dermatol 42:883–884 (May) 2000

FLUCONAZOLE
QT Prolongation, Torsades de Pointes

A 59-year-old inpatient with a Candida albicans infection in the ascitic fluid developed palpitations and polymorphic ventricular complexes (PVC's) after two days of intravenous and intraperitoneal fluconazole dosing. The patient was admitted for liver cirrhosis and peritonitis. Intravenous fluconazole was administered in doses of 400 to 800 mg daily for five weeks followed by intraperitoneal administration of 150 mg daily. Although EKGs were normal upon admission, after fluconazole dosing, QTc interval was prolonged (606 msec). Electrolyte and thyroid values were within normal ranges. However, serum fluconazole levels were elevated approximately eight to ten fold (216 mg/mL). Arrhythmias resolved and the QTc intervals normalized within three days and three weeks, respectively after fluconazole was stopped. All other medications remained the same.

The authors concluded that elevated fluconazole levels were responsible for QT prolongation and Torsades de pointes in this patient. They noted that intraperitoneal administration of fluconazole may increase systemic absorption and result in increased serum concentrations.

Wassmann S et al (Univ Cologne, 50924 Cologne, Germany) Long QT syndrome and torsades de pointes in a patient receiving fluconazole. Ann Intern Med 13(10):797 (Nov 16) 1999 (letter)

MICONAZOLE (VAGINAL) AND WARFARIN
Interaction: Increased Anticoagulation Effect
(First Report*)

A 53-year-old woman, previously stabilized on warfarin therapy (45 mg/week) developed bruising on her legs and arms approximately three days after starting vaginal miconazole therapy (200 mg suppositories) for a yeast infection. The only other concurrent medication was mexiletine (200 mg three times daily) for ventricular tachycardia. Prior to miconazole therapy, INRs were stabilized at a mean of 2.69. However, INRs taken on the third and last day of miconazole therapy were significantly elevated (9.77) until warfarin dosing was held for 24 hours (6.93). Rechallenge with miconazole therapy was required due to a persistent vaginal infection. Miconazole vaginal suppositories were restarted at 100 mg daily for seven days. Reduced warfarin dosing (32.5 mg/week) during concurrent therapy resulted in INRs within previous ranges (3.27). After miconazole therapy was discontinued, warfarin dosing was increased to previous dosage levels with subsequent therapeutic INRs.

Approximately one year later, a repeat seven day course of miconazole (100 mg) vaginal therapy was required due to another yeast infection. Despite a 19% reduction in warfarin dosing during concurrent therapy, INRs increased to 7.13. However, evidence of clinical bleeding was absent. INRs returned to 3.72 when warfarin was held for two days.

The authors noted that this is the first published case report of a drug interaction with vaginal miconazole therapy and warfarin. Although only a small amount of vaginal miconazole is thought to reach the systemic circulation, the authors proposed that this drug interfered with previously stable warfarin therapy. Possible proposed mechanisms of action included either a decrease in warfarin clearance or an increase in the plasma free fraction portion of warfarin. The authors encouraged clinicians to be aware of this potentially significant drug interaction and to adjust the warfarin dose accordingly.

Thirton DJG et al (Farquhar Zanetti LA: Anticoagulation Clin Henry Ford Health System, 3500 Fifteen Mile Rd, Sterling Heights, MI 48310) Potentiation of warfarin's hypothrombinemic effect with miconazole vaginal suppositories. Pharmacotherapy 20(1): 98–99 (Jan) 2000

ANTIVIRALS
ANTIRETROVIRAL THERAPY
Curly Hair, Lipodystrophy

A 48-year-old HIV positive patient developed curly hair and peripheral lipoatrophy approximately 1.5 years after starting lamivudine, stavudine, and indinavir therapy (dosages not provided). Other concurrent medications included glucocorticoids and mineralocorticoid supplementation for adrenal insufficiency. Despite the development of successful surgical and radiation treatment of spinocellular epithelioma, his viral load remained undetectable and his hair remained curly.

The authors noted that hair changes occurred in this patient during antiretroviral therapy and prior to the clinical manifestations of the anal tumor. They noted that lipodystrophy has been reported with protease inhibitors and hair pattern changes may be related to protease inhibition of cytoplasmic retinoic acid binding protein type 1.

Colebunders R et al (Instit Tropical Med, Dept Clin Sciences, Nationalestraat 155, B-2000 Antwerp, Belgium; e-mail:bcoleb@itg.be) Curly hair and lipodystrophy as a result of highly active antiretroviral treatment. Arch Dermatol 136:1064–1065 (Aug) 2000 (letter)

ANTIRETROVIRALS AND METHYLPREDNISOLONE
Immunosuppression, Legal Action

A 39-year-old HIV positive patient received concurrent therapy with methylprednisolone (large unspecified doses), 14 HIV medications, and six diarrhea medications. Methylprednisolone doses were prescribed for a period of six months. The patient was instructed to purchase medications at a pharmacy co-owned by the prescriber. The plaintiff alleged that the chronic administration of methylprednisolone was contraindicated with concurrent HIV medications and caused immunosuppression, thus, causing the development of resistance and shortened life expectancy. A settlement of one million dollars was reached prior to the beginning of the trial.

M Keifhaver vs LR Anisman, Pride Medical Services PC & Pride Medical, Inc. Use of steroid solumedrol for six months while taking multiple HIV medications contraindicated—weakened immune system—$1 million Georgia settlement. Med Malpractice Verdicts, Settlements & Experts 16(8):25 (Aug) 2000

ABACAVIR SULFATE
Fatal Hypersensitivity Reactions

On January 25, 2000 the manufacturer of abacavir (Glaxo Wellcome) contacted health professionals regarding newly revised warnings of the product package insert. Specifically, the information was about fatal hypersensitivity reactions in patients presenting with respiratory symptoms. Symptoms typically include fever, rash, nausea, vomiting, diarrhea and/or abdominal pain. Patients with fatal hypersensitivity reactions to this agent were initially diagnosed with an acute respiratory illness such as pneumonia, bronchitis or flu-like illness. Later during the course of treatment it was recognized that this syndrome was a hypersensitivity reaction to abacavir. Unfortunately, delayed diagnosis may result in continued administration of abacavir, worsening the reaction. Respiratory symptoms have been present in approximately 20% of the patients with abacavir hypersensitivity reactions. In addition, clinicians are encouraged to stop abacavir therapy if an illness cannot be clearly differentiated as a pulmonary infection or hypersensitivity reaction in patients receiving therapy.

Important safety information—fatal hypersensitivity reactions, respiratory symptoms, and ziagen. Glaxo-Wellcome Pharmaceuticals (Jan 25) 2000. (http://www.fda.gov/medwatch/safety/2000/ziagen3.pdf)

ABACAVIR
Severe Hypersensitivity Reactions, FDA Advisory

On July 27, 2000, the manufacturer (Glaxo Wellcome) of abacavir notified health professionals regarding the potential for severe or fatal hypersensitivity reactions that can occur within hours after reintroduction in patients with a history of previous hypersensitivity reactions. In the majority of reported cases, hypersensitivity was not recognized prior to stopping the drug and the discontinuation of abacavir therapy occurred for nonhypersensitivity causes (e.g., drug supply, treatment of other disease states). Although in most cases, there was a short onset of the reaction after reintroduction of the drug, in a few reports the onset was as long as a few days to weeks. It is recommended that once abacavir therapy is stopped, the reason for drug withdrawal should be re-evaluated prior to reintroduction. In addition, the patient should be counseled regarding potential hypersensitivity reactions, and the drug prescribed with caution and in situations where medical care is available for potentially serious reactions.

Hypersensitivity reactions with abacavir. (Jul) 2000. http://www.fda.gov/medwatch/safety/2000/ziagen.htm

AMANTADINE vs RIMANTADINE
CNS Adverse Events

In a retrospective cohort study, CNS adverse events were monitored in 156 nursing home patients (mean age: 83.7 yrs) who received sequential therapy with amantadine and rimantadine during the 1997–1998 influenza season. The average duration of therapy in all patients was 20.6 days and 26.3 days for amantadine and rimantadine, respectively. In patients with CNS adverse events, however, therapy duration was significantly shorter (10.9 days and 16.3 days). In contrast, patients who did not develop adverse events were able to take the medications for longer periods (22.6 vs 26.5 days). Most patients were receiving one other CNS active medication (67%) and approximately one-fourth (26%) were taking several CNS medications. In the amantadine group there was a significantly higher rate of patients with any adverse event (18.6% vs 1.9%), and an adverse event requiring drug withdrawal (17.3% vs 1.9%). Other adverse events with a higher incidence in the amantadine group included agitation (4.5% vs 1.3%), confusion (10.3% vs 0.6%), hallucinations (3.9% vs 0%), lethargy (1.3% vs 0.6%), seizures (1.3% vs 0%) and tremors (1.9% vs 0%). Risk factors for CNS adverse effects in this population included males, reduced creatinine clearance, and use of amantadine.

The authors concluded that amantadine was associated with a significantly higher rate of central nervous adverse events than rimantadine in this study population, and is often the cause for discontinuation of the drug. The authors also noted that possible causes of this difference could not be identified, as this was a retrospective study.

Keyser LA et al (Bertino JS, Clin Pharmacy Serv, Clin Pharmacology Res Center, Bassett Healthcare, 1 Atwell Rd, Cooperstown, NY 13326; e-mail:jbertino@ iex.net) Comparison of central nervous system adverse effects of amantadine and rimantadine used a sequential prophylaxis of influenza A in elderly nursing home patients. Arch Intern Med 160:1485–1488 (May 22) 2000

AMPRENAVIR AND KETOCONAZOLE
Interaction: Increased Serum Concentrations

In a randomized, open-label, tri-period crossover study, 12 healthy male volunteers (median age: 23 years) received a single dose of either amprenavir (1200 mg) or ketoconazole (400 mg) alone or in combination. Each dose was separated by 14 days. Combination therapy resulted in increased AUCs for both amprenavir (31%: 29.5 vs 22.0 mcg.hr/mL) and ketoconazole (44%: 49.5 vs 35.2 mcg.hr/mL) as compared to each drug alone. Significant increases also occurred in ketoconazole's peak concentrations (19%: 8.5 vs 7.3 mcg/mL) and half-life (23%: 2.3 vs 1.9 hrs). Significant decreases were noted in amprenavir's peak concentration (16%: 0.84 vs 1.0 mcg/mL) and half-life (16%: 8.7 vs 6.6 hrs).

The authors observed that coadministration of ketoconazole and amprenavir resulted in significant increases in the AUC for both agents. The most likely mechanisms by which ketoconazole may increase amprenavir's AUC include increased absorption via CYP3A gastrointestinal inhibition or increased bioavailability via P-glycoprotein inhibition. Further multidose, long term studies are required before the clinical significance can be determined.

Polk RE et al (Dept Pharmacy, Virginia Commonwealth University/Med Coll Virginia Campus, PO Box 980533 MCV, Richmond, VA 23298) Pharmacokinetic interaction between ketoconazole and amprenavir after single doses in healthy men. Pharmacotherapy 19(12):1378–1384 (Dec) 1999

AMPRENAVIR
Propylene Glycol Content and Potential Risks

In May 2000, the FDA and manufacturer of amprenavir notified health professionals regarding the potential risks associated with a large amount of excipient (propylene glycol) in the oral solution. Some patients may not be able to adequately metabolize and eliminate propylene glycol, potentially causing accumulation and possible toxicities. Patients with reduced metabolic activity and amprenavir use who would be contraindicated include infants, children less than four years of age, pregnant women, patients with renal or hepatic impairment, and patients taking metronidazole or disulfiram. Although there have been no reactions related to this issue to date, the product labeling will reflect notices regarding this potential problem.

Potential safety concerns with large amounts of propylene glycol in Agenerase (amprenavir) oral solution. (http://www.fda.gov/medwatch/safety/2000/agener.htm) (May) 2000

INDINAVIR
Crystalluria

A 25-year-old HIV positive patient developed flank pain and dysuria approximately six weeks after starting indinavir (800 mg every eight hours). Concurrent medication included lamivudine (150 mg twice daily), zidovudine (300 mg twice daily), sertraline (50 mg daily), and zolpidem (10 mg nightly). Further evaluation revealed hematuria and crystalluria, which persisted despite increased fluid intake (up to 48 ounces daily) for an additional week. After nelfinavir (250 mg five tablets every 12 hours) replaced indinavir therapy, symptoms and crystalluria resolved within one week.

The authors theorized that indinavir was responsible for crystalluria in this patient. No mechanism of action was provided.

Hachey DM et al (Force RW, Idaho State Univ, Campus Box 8357, Pocatello, ID 83209; e-mail:Force@otc.isu.edu) Indinavir crystalluria in an HIV positive man. Ann Pharmacother 34:403 (Mar) 2000

INDINAVIR
Crystalluria

In a one year prospective study, 54 asymptomatic HIV-positive patients (mean age: 42.8 yrs) were monitored for urinary complications during indinavir therapy (800 mg every eight hours) for a mean duration of 51.2 weeks. Routine urinalyses were performed at a mean of 11.2 times/patient. Dipstick urine analysis was clear for most urine samples (82%) during indinavir therapy, including negative results for glucose (96%), ketones (96.5%), blood (89.8%), nitrites (98%), and leukocytes (93.9%). Although specific gravity was at least 1.025 in approximately 66% of the samples, results did not differ from baseline. In contrast, crystalluria, which was absent at baseline measurement, occurred in 11% at week two, in 28% by week four, and in 25% till the end of the study. Intermittent crystalluria occurred in most patients (31) but almost one third (18) never developed crystalluria during therapy. Crystalluria was more frequently associated with high urine pH but data.

The authors concluded that most patients are not adequately hydrated during indinavir therapy, increasing the risk of crystal formation. They recommended that patients on indinavir therapy should increase water intake, particularly at the time of dosing and four hours post dosing. They also proposed that increased specific gravity may be a potential risk factor for the development of crystalluria.

Gagnon RF et al. (Div Nephrol, Rm L4-516, Montreal Gen Hosp, 1650 Cedar Ave, Montreal, Quebec, Canada H3G 1A4; e-mail:raymonde.gagnon@muhc.mcgill.ca) Prospective study of urinalysis abnormalities in HIV positive individuals treated with indinavir. Am J Kidney Diseases 36(3):507–515 (Sep) 2000

INDINAVIR AND ST. JOHN'S WORT
Interaction: Decreased Indinavir Concentrations, FDA Advisory

On February 10th, 2000 the FDA published a public health advisory regarding a recent NIH study which demonstrated a significant drug interaction between St. John's wort (hypericum perforatum) and indinavir. Concurrent administration resulted in decreased indinavir concentrations possibly related to cytochrome P450 isoenzyme induction. The FDA recommended that St. John's wort should not be used concurrently with any of the currently marketed protease inhibitors or nonnucleoside transcriptase inhibitor antiretrovirals as suboptimal plasma concentrations may reduce virologic response and promote resistance. The FDA is working with manufacturers of the antiretrovirals to revise product labeling to include these new recommendations.

FDA Public Health Advisory. Risk of drug interactions with St. John's wort and indinavir and other drugs. (Feb 10) 2000. http://www.fda. gov/cder/drug/advisory/stjwort.htm

INDINAVIR AND ST. JOHN'S WORT
Interaction: Decreased Indinavir Concentrations

In an open label study, eight healthy male volunteers (age range: 29 to 50 yrs) received indinavir alone (800 mg) every eight hours for four doses. After monotherapy plasma concentrations were obtained, St. John's wort (300 mg three times daily) was administered with meals for 14 days. Four doses of indinavir (800 mg every eight hours on an empty stomach) therapy were administered during the last two days of St. John's wort therapy. Although time to maximum indinavir concentrations were unchanged with or without St. John's wort administration (1.1 hrs), the mean AUC at eight hours was decreased by 57% when administered with the herbal product (30.8 mcg.hr/mL vs 12.3 mcg.hr/mL). Concurrent administration also resulted in reduced indinavir concentrations at eight hours by a range of 49% to 99%. Mean maximum concentrations were also reduced (12.3 mcg/mL to 8.9 mcg/mL).

The authors concluded that indinavir plasma concentrations are significantly reduced by concurrent St. John's wort therapy most likely via

CYP3A4 isoenzyme induction. Because other antiretrovirals are also metabolized by the same isoenzyme system, they recommended that these combinations be avoided until further information is available.

Piscitelli SC et al (Dept Pharmacy, Warren G Magnuson Clin Center & Lab of Immunoregulation, NIH, Bethesda, MD 20892; e-mail:spisc@nih.gov) Indinavir concentrations and St. John's wort. Lancet 355:547 (Feb 12) 2000 (letter)

PROTEASE INHIBITORS
Hyperprolactinemia

Four cases of galactorrhea and hyperprolactinemia were reported in female patients taking protease inhibitors.

Patient 1: A patient (no age provided) developed gynecomastia within one month after starting an antiretroviral regimen consisting of ritonavir, saquinavir, lamivudine, and stavudine for HIV infection. Galactorrhea and hyperprolactinemia (4130 mU/L) also were noted. The only concurrent medication included cotrimoxazole. Symptoms resolved within two weeks after ritonavir and saquinavir were discontinued and prolactin levels returned to normal ranges within one month.

Patient 2: A patient (no age provided) developed galactorrhea and hyperprolactinemia (1027 mU/L) approximately 12.5 months after starting lamivudine, stavudine, and indinavir for HIV-1 infection. Concurrent medications included cotrimoxazole, norethistrerone, and fluoxetine, which were started four months prior to the adverse event. Symptoms persisted despite the discontinuation of fluoxetine. However, symptoms resolved once nelfinavir was substituted for indinavir.

Patient 3: A female patient (no age provided) developed breast tenderness and galactorrhea after starting postexposure prophylaxis with zidovudine, lamivudine, and indinavir. Concurrent medications included domperidone (later switched to metoclopramide), ciprofloxacin, azithromycin, metronidazole, fluconazole and post-coital contraception. Symptoms resolved after the antiviral regimen was discontinued.

Patient 4: A female patient (no age specified) developed galactorrhea and breast enlargement with hyperprolactinemia (1091 mU/L) after starting zidovudine, lamivudine, indinavir as post exposure prophylaxis therapy for a needlestick injury. Symptoms resolved and prolactin levels returned to baseline within three weeks after prophylaxis regimens were discontinued.

The authors suggested that protease inhibitors alone or in combination with other select drugs (e.g., dopamine agonists) may have caused hyperprolactinemia in these patients.

Hutchinson J et al. (Med & Emergency Directorate, Infection & Immunity Specialty Group, St. Bartholomew's and the London NHS Trust, West Smithfield, London EC1A 7 BE, UK) Galactorrhea and hyperprolactinemia associated with protease inhibitors. Lancet 356:1003–1004 (Sep 16) 2000 (letter)

PROTEASE INHIBITORS
Hyperglycemia

In a retrospective chart review, 121 HIV urban minority patients who had taken protease inhibitors during a one year period were identified. Four of these patients had been previously diagnosed with diabetes and were excluded from the analysis. Of the remaining 117, seven (6%) developed new onset diabetes mellitus during therapy. The mean onset of symptoms (polydipsia and polyuria) occurred approximately 11 weeks after the initiation of therapy. All of the patients who developed diabetes received indinavir in combination with lamivudine and zidovudine or stavudine. Two patients required hospitalization for nonketotic hyperosmolar state. None of the patients had ketonuria, but all of the patients had increased serum triglycerides (mean: 638 mg/dL) compared to baseline levels (mean: 226 mg/dL). In patients who did not develop symptomatic diabetes, mean glucose levels were significantly higher when compared to baseline (100 mg/dL vs 95 mg/dL).

The authors concluded that urban minority HIV patients receiving combination antiretroviral therapy including a protease inhibitor may be at increased risk for developing hyperglycemia and diabetes. They also recommended that risk factors for diabetes should be identified prior to initiation of therapy and close blood glucose monitoring employed during therapy.

Dever LL et al. (Med Service (111), VA New Jersey Health Care System, 385 Tremont Ave, East Orange, NJ 07018; email:dever.lisa@east-orange.va.gov) Hyperglycemia associated with protease inhibitors in an urban HIV infected minority patient population. Ann Pharmacother 34:580–584 (May) 2000

RITONAVIR AND FENTANYL
Interaction: Decreased Fentanyl Clearance,
Increased Half-life

In a double blinded, placebo controlled crossover study, 12 health subjects received either oral ritonavir or placebo for three days. Ritanovir was dosed at 200 mg three times daily the first day, followed by 300 mg three times daily on the second day. On the third morning, the last dose of ritonavir or placebo was given. On day two, intravenous fentanyl (5 mcg/kg) was administered over two minutes. Naloxone (0.1 mg) was also administered prior to and with fentanyl to prevent sedative and respiratory effects typically associated with fentanyl. Eleven subjects completed the study; one patient withdrew as a result of nausea and vomiting. Ritonavir reduced fentanyl clearance by 67% (15.6 to 5.2 mL/min/kg) accompanied by increases in AUC (4.8 to 8.8 ng/mL) and fentanyl half-life (9.4 vs 20.1 hrs). Eight of the 11 patients completing the study reported nausea.

The authors concluded that ritonavir inhibited the metabolism of fentanyl, possibly via the CYP3A4 isoenzyme system. They also suggested that decreases in fentanyl elimination may increase the risks of respiratory depression in patients receiving this combination.

Olkkola KT et al (Dept Anesth, Toolo Hosp, Helsinki Univ Central Hosp, PO Box 266, FIN-00029 HYKS, Finland) Ritonavir's role in reducing fentanyl clearance and prolonging its half-life. Anesthesiology 91:681–685 (Sep) 1999

RITONAVIR AND MEPERIDINE
Interaction: Decreased Meperidine and Increased Normeperidine Concentrations

In an open-label, crossover, pharmacokinetic study, eight healthy volunteers received a single oral dose of meperidine (50 mg). Two days later they started ritonavir therapy (500 mg twice daily) for 13 days. On day 10 another single dose of meperidine was administered. After ritonavir administration the mean meperidine AUC was decreased by 67% (172.3 vs 522.7 ng.hr/mL) and peak concentrations were also decreased by approximately 40% (51.1 vs 125.8 ng/mL). However time to peak concentration was unaffected (1.2 vs 1.5 hrs). In contrast, mean normeperidine AUC was increased by 47% after concurrent ritonavir administration (361.7 vs 246 ng.hr/mL), as were peak concentrations (38.6 vs 20.6 ng/mL). Time to peak concentration was decreased after ritonavir administration (2.7 vs 4 hrs).

The authors suggested that increased normeperidine concentrations reflect an induction of CYP-mediated metabolism via ritonavir. They proposed that CYP1A2 might be the predominant isoenzyme responsible for meperidine metabolism. Another theory suggests that simultaneous induction/inhibition of the competing metabolic pathways results in an overall net induction effect. Although the risk of increased meperidine side effects during concurrent ritonavir therapy appears low, the risk of normeperidine accumulation may be increased.

Piscitelli SC et al (Clinical Center Pharmacy Dept, Bldg. 10, Room 1N257, NIH, Bethesda, MD 20892) The effect of ritonavir on the pharmacokinetics of meperidine and normeperidine. Pharmacotherapy 20(5):549–553 (May) 2000

RITONAVIR AND METHADONE
Interaction: Decreased Methadone Effect

A 51-year-old patient, previously stabilized in a methadone program (90 mg daily) for two years, was hospitalized for withdrawal symptoms, which began approximately 5.5 hours prior to admission. Ritonavir (400 mg twice daily), saquinavir (400 mg twice daily), and stavudine (40 mg twice daily) had recently been started seven days earlier. Other chronic medications included TMP/SMX (160/800 mg every other day), fosinopril (20 mg daily), and cimetidine (400 mg twice daily). Liver function tests were consistent with baseline studies, with the exception of an elevated gamma-glutamyl transferase (191 U/L). Methadone levels at the time of admission were 210 ng/mL. The patient was stabilized on increased methadone doses during hospitalization (100 mg daily) and post discharge (130 mg daily).

The authors suggested that ritonavir was most likely responsible for withdrawal symptoms in this patient as a result of decreased methadone serum levels via hepatic isoenzyme induction. They encouraged clinicians to be aware of this possible interaction and recommended that formal clinical studies be performed.

Geletko SM & Erickson AD. Decreased methadone effect after ritonavir initiation. Pharmacotherapy 20(1):93–94 (Jan) 2000

RITONAVIR
Hepatotoxicity in Hepatitis C or B Infection

The incidence of severe hepatotoxicity during antiretroviral therapy was examined in a prospective cohort study of 298 patients who received protease inhibitors in combination therapy. Chronic hepatitis C and B virus infections were present in 52% and 3% of the patients, respectively. Overall, severe hepatotoxicity was observed in 10.4% (31/298) of the patients monitored with the highest incidence of toxicity associated with ritonavir therapy (30%). Treatment groups not associated with significant risk included nucleoside analogs (5.7%), nelfinavir (5.9%), saquinavir (5.9%) and indinavir (6.8%). Patients with hepatitis C or B infections were also at risk of hepatotoxicity.

The authors concluded that the use of ritonavir increased the risk of severe hepatotoxicity and may be more common in patients with chronic viral hepatitis. However, they did not recommend withholding protease inhibitor therapy in patients with such infections.

Sulkowski MS et al (Div Infectious Dis, Johns Hopkins Univ, Sch Med, 1830 E Monument St, Suite 450C, Baltimore MD 21287; e-mail:msulkowskis@jhmi.edu) Hepatotoxicity associated with antiretroviral therapy in adults infected with human immunodeficiency virus and the role of hepatitis C or B virus infection. JAMA 283:74–80 (Jan 5) 2000

SAQUINAVIR
Hypoglycemia

A 49-year-old HIV positive patient who was also a type 2 diabetic developed dizziness approximately six weeks after his antiviral regimen was changed. Insulin requirements prior to the change were 40 units daily (human 70/30) and resulted in blood glucose values between 80 to 140 mg/dL. Previous antivirals included zidovudine, lamivudine and nelfinavir. The new antiviral regimen consisted of stavudine (40 mg twice daily), didanosine (200 mg twice daily), and saquinavir (1200 mg three times daily). Eight weeks after the regimen change the patient was admitted to the emergency room for a syncopal episode. At the time of admission, the patient was severely hypoglycemic (blood glucose: 24 mg/dL). Despite an increase in daily insulin dosages (20 units daily) the patient continued to have dizziness episodes related to hypoglycemia. Eventually the insulin was discontinued. Other causes for hypoglycemia were not identified.

The authors suggested that the addition of saquinavir to this patient's antiviral regimen was responsible for hypoglycemia. Although they cited similar episodes reported in the medical literature a mechanism of action was not provided.

Zimhony O & Stein D (Albert Einstein Coll Med, Bronx, NY 10461) Saquinavir induced hypoglycemia in type 2 diabetes. Ann Intern Med 131:980 (Dec 21) 1999 (letter)

VALACYCLOVIR
Thrombotic Thrombocytopenic Purpura

A 48-year-old HIV patient was hospitalized with fever and malaise. Chronic medications at the time of hospitalization included lamivudine, ritonavir, saquinavir, stavudine, and valacyclovir (500 mg twice daily). Upon admission, abnormal laboratory values included platelet count (8×10^9/L), hemoglobin (83 g/L), lactate dehydrogenase (5737 U/L), and serum haptoglobin (0.02 g/L). Bone marrow aspirate also revealed mild erythroid hyperplasia with a normal number of megakaryocytes. Serological screenings for infectious etiologies (e.g., hepatitis, syphilis) were negative. Treatment included intravenous methylprednisolone (240 mg daily), plasma infusions (30 mL/kg) and intravenous immunoglobulin (20 grams) after cutaneous purpura developed. Despite treatment the patient became confused and experienced a stroke. Several plasma exchanges were also performed over a five period with a gradual improvement in neurological symptoms, platelet counts and hemoglobin values. After 45 days of hospitalization the patient was discharged. Laboratory values documented at this time included hemoglobin (110 g/L), platelet count (146×10^9/L), and creatinine (77 umol/L). No recurrence of thrombotic thrombocytopenic purpura occurred during a one year follow up period.

The authors suggested that this case of thrombotic thrombocytopenic purpura was most likely caused by valacyclovir but recognized that HIV status may have also been the causal factor. A mechanism of action was not provided.

Rivaud E et al. (Suresnes, France) Valacyclovir hydrochloride therapy and thrombotic thrombocytopenic purpura in an HIV infected patient. Arch Intern Med 160:1705–1706 (Jun 12) 2000

ZANAMIVIR
Respiratory Distress

A 63-year-old patient with chronic obstructive pulmonary disease developed acute respiratory difficulty immediately after each zanamivir inhalation prescribed for suspected influenza. After only three days of zanamivir therapy, he was hospitalized with respiratory distress, hypoxia and leukocytosis (14,400/mm^3). A chest x-ray revealed mild pulmonary edema with emphysematous changes. Symptoms improved with bronchodilators, corticosteroids and antibiotics with patient discharge after three days of hospitalization.

The authors concluded that respiratory distress was associated with zanamivir use in this patient. Although an exact mechanism of action was not provided, the authors noted that manufacturer guidelines for zanamivir recommend that the drug be stopped if bronchospasm occurs or respiratory function deteriorates after drug use. In addition, patients with underlying lung disease should have ready access to inhaled bronchodilators if needed. This drug should be used with caution in patients with underlying lung disease.

Williamson JC et al (Wake Forest Univ Baptist Med Center, Winston-Salem, NC 27157) Respiratory distress associated with zanamivir. N Engl J Med 342:661–662 (Mar 2) 2000 (letter)

CEPHALOSPORINS
CEFAZOLIN
Fever

An adult inpatient (no age provided) developed a fever within 24 hours post-sialadenectomy. Post-operative medications included cefazolin (1 gram every eight hours), meperidine (50 mg as needed every four hours) and promethazine (25 mg every four hours as needed). Temperature spikes occurred in the morning and evening for two days postoperatively despite negative urine, blood and sputum cultures. Body temperature continued to decline after antibiotic discontinuation, reaching normal ranges by post-operative day four.

The authors concluded that the lack of infection and resolution of fever post cefazolin withdrawal indicated that cefazolin was responsible for this patient's fever.

Homrighausen J et al (207 Sparks Ave, Suite 205, Jeffersonville, IN 47130) Drug related fever due to cephazolin: a case report. J Oral Maxillofac Surg 57:1141–1143 (Sep) 1999

CEFDINIR
Red Stools

Two cases of red stools related to oral cefdinir therapy were reported in two pediatric outpatients.

Patient 1: A six-year-old outpatient with bronchopulmonary dysplasia developed red stools within 48 hours after starting cefdinir for a lower respiratory tract infection, cough and fever. The cefdinir was administered through a button gastrostomy (125 mg/5 mL; no dosage provided). The patient was also receiving Neocate One Plus Formula. Symptoms of gastrointestinal distress (e.g., abdominal pain, vomiting, diarrhea) were absent. Screening tests for infectious etiologies or gastrointestinal bleeding were also negative. The red stools resolved after another antibiotic was substituted for cefdinir. No time frame for symptom resolution was provided.

Patient 2: A five-month-old outpatient developed red stools within 24 hours after starting cefdinir for an otitis media infection, which was refractory to several previous antibiotic regimens. Dosage information was not provided. The patient was also receiving Alimentum. Symptoms of gastrointestinal distress (e.g., abdominal pain, vomiting, diarrhea) were absent. Screening tests for infectious etiologies or gastrointestinal bleeding were also negative. The red stools resolved after the full course of cefdinir was completed. No time frame for symptom resolution was provided.

The authors concluded that cefdinir therapy was responsible for red stools in both these patients, possibly related to the formation of a nonabsorbable complex between a cefdinir byproduct and iron in the gastrointestinal tract. Both patients were receiving enteral formulas which contained iron. The authors recommended that cefdinir should be taken two hours before or after the iron supplements.

Nelson JS (Creighton Univ Sch Med, Midwest Allergy & Asthma Clin, Omaha, NE 68114) Red stools and Omnicef. J Pediatrics 136(6):853–854 (Jun) 2000

CEFOTETAN
Hemolysis

Three cases of cefotetan induced hemolysis were reported in three obstetric patients who had received the drug prophylactically during or immediately after a cesarean delivery.

Patient 1: A 37-year-old pregnant woman received a single dose of intravenous cefotetan (2 grams) during a cesarean delivery of twins. Thirteen days post delivery, she was rehospitalized with severe dyspnea and a reduced hematocrit (11%). Hemolysis as the cause of anemia was confirmed via positive agglutination results when red blood cells were combined with cefotetan. The patient's recovery was uneventful after treatment with transfusion of four units of packed red blood cells.

Patient 2: A 36-year-old pregnant woman received a single dose of intravenous cefotetan (2 grams) near the completion of a cesarean delivery of a healthy baby. Nine days post delivery, the patient had a reduced hematocrit (23%). A peripheral blood smear indicated hemolysis as the cause of anemia, which was confirmed via positive agglutination results when red blood cells were combined with cefotetan. The patient's recovery was uneventful after treatment with oral corticosteroids.

Patient 3: A 23-year-old pregnant woman received a single dose of intravenous cefotetan (2 grams) during a cesarean delivery of a healthy baby. Nine days post delivery, she was rehospitalized with fatigue, jaundice, and severe anemia (hematocrit: 8%). Hemolysis as the cause of anemia was confirmed via positive agglutination results when red blood cells were combined with cefotetan. The patient's recovery was uneventful after treatment with transfusion of four units of packed red blood cells and intravenous corticosteroids.

The authors concluded that cefotetan induced hemolytic anemia in these three patients after only a single dose administration. They recommended that first generation cephalosporins may be preferred as they are as effective as second or third generation cephalosporins and have a decreased risk of hemolytic anemia.

Naylor CS et al (Dept Obstetrics & Gynecology, Cedars Sinai Med Center, 9700 Beverly Blvd, Suite 3611, Los Angeles, CA 90048) Cefotetan induced hemolysis associated with antibiotic prophylaxis for cesarean delivery. Am J Obstet Gynecol 182:1427–1428 (Jul) 2000

CEFTAZIDIME AND VANCOMYCIN (INTRAVITREAL)
Ocular Precipitation

Two cases of precipitates are described after subconjunctival and intravitreous injections of vancomycin and ceftazidime.

Patient 1: A 17-year-old patient with post-traumatic eye inflammation developed dense yellow-white precipitates in the vitreous cavity immediately after subconjunctival and intravitreal injections of ceftazidime and vancomycin. Intravitreal concentrations for ceftazidime and vancomycin were 2.2 mg/0.1 mL and 1 mg/0.1 mL, respectively. Subconjunctival concentrations were 100 mg/0.5 mL and 25 mg/0.25 mL, respectively. Conjunctival precipitates were easily removed via ocular washings. Vitreous precipitates gradually resolved over a two month period without damaging vision.

Patient 2: A 44-year-old man with a post traumatic endophthalmitis developed dense yellow white precipitates in the vitreous cavity immediately after intravitreal injections of ceftazidime (2.2 mg/0.1 mL) and vancomycin

(1 mg/0.1 mL). Similar precipitates developed after subconjunctival injections with the same drugs. Vitreous opacities resolved over a two month period and vision stabilized at 20/30.

The authors simulated similar precipitates after injecting the drugs in a fresh pig's eye, confirming that the precipitation was due to the drug pH incompatibility. They advised against use of this intravitreal combination until further studies can confirm the interaction.

Lifshitz T et al (Dept Ophthalmol, Soroka Univ Med Center, Ben Gurion Univ Negev, POB 151, Beer Sheba 84101, Israel) Vancomycin and ceftazidime incompatibility upon intravitreal injection. Br J Ophthalmol 84:1117 (Jan) 2000 (letter)

CEFUROXIME
Lymphomatoid Hypersensitivity Reaction

An 84-year-old inpatient developed an erythematous and purpuric rash on the lower extremities within three days after starting intravenous cefuroxime (750 mg three times daily) for acute diverticulitis and septic shock. Other concurrent medications included intravenous metronidazole (500 mg every eight hours) and intravenous fluids. Treatment included topical flucinolone acetonide (0.00625%).

Screenings for non-drug etiologies were negative. A skin biopsy indicated a mixed dermal infiltrate of lymphoid cells and eosinophils. A histological examination revealed that the infiltrate was T cell rich with most large cells being CD30 positive. The rash subsided within 10 days after cefuroxime therapy was discontinued and did not recur during a 15 month follow-up period.

The authors concluded that this reaction was most aptly described as a lymphomatoid vascular reaction caused by an allergic response. The precise mechanism of this type of drug induced reaction is not clear but may be related to a delayed type hypersensitivity reaction.

Saeed SAM et al. (Bazza M, Dept Dermatol, Walsall Manor Hosp, Walsall West Hosp, Walsall West Midlands WS2 9 PS, UK) Cefuroxime induced lymphomatoid hypersensitivity reaction. Postgrad Med J 76:577–579 (Sep) 2000

MACROLIDES
CLARITHROMYCIN AND OMEPRAZOLE
Interaction: Omeprazole Concentrations Increased

In a double blinded, randomized cross-over study, 21 healthy volunteers received either placebo or clarithromycin (400 mg twice daily) for three days followed by a morning dose of omeprazole (20 mg) with clarithromycin (400 mg) or placebo. CYP2C19 genotype status was determined, with six subjects classified as homozygous extensive metabolizers,

11 subjects classified as heterozygous extensive metabolizers and four subjects as poor metabolizers. In all groups, plasma omeprazole levels were significantly increased (greater than two fold) during concurrent clarithromycin administration. AUC omeprazole values were highest in the poor metabolizer group (13,098.6 ng/hr/mL) as compared to the heterozygous extensive metabolizers (2,110.4 ng/hr/mL) and homozygous extensive metabolizers (813.1 ng/hr/mL). Mean AUC values for omeprazole-sulfone (a metabolite of omeprazole via CYP3A4 isoenzyme) were also highest in the poor metabolizer group when compared to the two extensive metabolizer groups (3,304.2 vs 435.3 vs 188.6). In contrast, AUC mean values for 5-hydroxy omeprazole were lowest in the poor metabolizer group (220.5 vs 1016.8 vs 946.0).

The authors concluded that omeprazole increased plasma concentrations of clarithromycin in all genotypes groups, but caused greater increases in the CYP2C19 poor metabolizer group. They also suggested that the combination use of these agents to treat H. pylori ulcers may result in higher eradication rates because of increased plasma levels.

Furuta T et al (First Dept of Med, Hamamatsu Uni Sch Med, 3600, Handa-cho, Hamamatsu, 431-3192, Japan) Effects of clarithromycin on the metabolism of omeprazole in relation to CYP2C19 genotype status in humans. Clin Pharmacol & Ther 66: 265–274 (Sep) 1999

CLARITHROMYCIN AND ITRACONAZOLE
Interaction: Increased Clarithromycin Concentrations

Three case reports describing a potential interaction with itraconazole and clarithromycin are provided below.

Patient 1: A 55-year-old man with HIV infection and hospitalized for suspected pulmonary Mycobacterium avium complex (MAC) received clarithromycin (500 mg daily), ethambutol (800 mg daily), levofloxacin (500 mg daily), itraconazole (100 mg twice daily), digoxin (dosage not provided), ibuprofen (400 mg every six hours) and intravenous gentamicin (225 mg daily). After two days of therapy both clarithromycin and itraconazole parent serum levels were above expected values (15.53 mcg/mL and 0.97 mcg/mL). In addition, the serum levels of the clarithromycin metabolite, 14-OH clarithromycin was also higher than expected (1.38 mcg/mL) as was the parent:metabolite ratio (11.25 vs 3). Although clarithromycin levels remained elevated no clinical adverse effects were observed. The antibiotic was stopped on day five when MAC was not confirmed.

Patient 2: A 38-year-old woman with HIV infection was hospitalized for cystic fibrosis and pulmonary MAC and aspergillosis infections. Medications during hospitalization included ethambutol (1 gram daily), clofazamine (100 mg daily), clarithromycin (500 mg daily), itraconazole

(200 mg twice daily), ibuprofen (600 mg every four to six hours as needed) and vitamins A, D, E and K. After four days of concurrent therapy with itraconazole, serum levels of clarithromycin and the 14-OH metabolite were increased (2.93 and 3.71 mcg/mL, respectively) when measured at three hours post dosing. Parent compound levels (clarithromycin) were further increased after 11 days of concurrent therapy (9.58 mcg/mL). In addition, itraconazole levels were also elevated at 1.51 mcg/mL. However, within one day after itraconazole was discontinued, clarithromycin levels decreased to 4.79 mcg/mL. The patient did not experience any adverse clinical effects attributed to increased serum concentrations.

Patient 3: A 45-year-old woman with HIV and chronic MAC pulmonary disease exhibited increased clarithromycin and itraconazole serum concentrations during concurrent therapy. Medications included ethambutol (900 mg daily), ciprofloxacin (500 mg daily), clarithromycin (500 mg daily), itraconazole (200 mg twice daily), amikacin, albuterol and sodium docusate (dosages not provided). After five days of concurrent therapy, serum clarithromycin levels were elevated at three and seven hours post dosing (11.04 and 11.9 mcg/mL). In addition the parent:metabolite ratio was also greater than expected (6.8 vs 3).

The authors concluded that itraconazole increased the serum concentrations of clarithromycin by 37% to 122% higher than expected values. They suggested that there is a bi-directional interaction between the drugs, possibly caused by both their inhibitory activities on the CYP3A4 hepatic isoenzyme system. Although none of the patients experienced adverse events related to increased serum concentrations, the authors suggested that further clinical study is needed before these two drugs can be clearly established to be administered safely together.

Auclair B et al (Peloquin CA: Pharmacokinetics Lab, Rm D-106, National Jewish Med & Research Center, 1400 Jackson St, Denver, CO 80206) Potential interaction between itraconazole and clarithromycin. Pharmacotherapy 19:1439–1444 (Dec) 1999

ERYTHROMYCIN
Infantile Hypertrophic Pyloric Stenosis

In March 1999, seven cases of infantile hypertrophic pyloric stenosis (IHPS) occurred during a two week period. All the cases were among 200 infants who had received a prophylactic oral regimen of erythromycin in the same hospital after a possible exposure to pertussis. To examine the possibility of a causal relationship between the drug and IHPS, a retrospective cohort study was performed in 282 infants born in the same hospital during a two-month period (January through February 1999). Of these cases, approximately half (157/282) received oral erythromycin, including the ethylsuccinate (n = 83) and estolate (n = 59). There was no difference in the risk of IHPS when the type of erythromycin used was examined. Infants who did not develop IHPS while on erythromycin had a mean age of 14.1 days and received the drug for a mean of 12.2 days (range 1 to 21 days). The seven IHPS cases had a mean age of 9.3 days and received erythromycin for a mean of 13.3 days (range: 10 to 18 days). All IHPS patients developed initial symptoms of either vomiting or excessive irritability.

The authors concluded that this data suggests a possible causal relationship between erythromycin and the cluster of IHPS cases. They recommended that prescribers should inform parents about the possible risk of developing IHPS with erythromycin therapy.

Hypertrophic pyloric stenosis in infants following pertussis prophylaxis with erythromycin—Knoxville, Tennessee, 1999. Morbidity Mortality Weekly Report (MMWR) 48(49):1117–1120 (Dec 17) 1999 (http://www.cdc.gov/epo/mmwr/preview/mmwrhtml/mm4849a1.htm)

MISCELLANEOUS
BACITRACIN (NASAL PACKING)
Anaphylaxis

A 48-year-old man developed an anaphylactic reaction within seconds after a latex glove finger filled with Vaseline gauze and coated with bacitracin was inserted into his right nostril after an otherwise uneventful septorhinoplasty. Initially, latex allergy was suspected, and nasal packing was immediately removed. After anesthesia emergence, the patient remained intubated in an intensive care setting for two days due to facial and upper airway edema. Upon a post-discharge evaluation, the patient indicated that he experienced nasal swelling and irritation after nasal application of an ointment containing polymixin B and bacitracin. The reaction resolved once the ointment was removed. Epicutaneous skin prick testing revealed positive reactions to bacitracin but not latex, polymixin, or control solutions (cefazolin and saline).

Based on the skin prick testing results, the authors concluded that bacitracin was responsible for this patient's anaphylactic reaction during surgery. They also noted that bacitracin use should be reconsidered because of this risk.

Gall R et al (Bell DD: St. Boniface Gen Hosp, D2020, 409 Tache Ave, Winnipeg, Manitoba, Canada R2H 2A6; e-mail:deanbell@compuserve.com) Intraoperative anaphylactic shock from bacitracin nasal packing after septorhinoplasty. An-esthesiology 91(5):1545–1547 (Nov) 1999

QUINUPRISTIN-DALFOPRISTIN
Hyponatremia

A 67-year-old inpatient with small cell carcinoma developed severe hyponatremia within one week after starting quinupristin-dalfopristin

(Quin/Dalf) therapy (7.5 mg/kg every eight hours) for vancomycin resistant E. faecium. Previous therapy prior to hospitalization included three cycles of chemotherapy with etoposide, cyclophosphamide, and adriamycin. Concurrent therapy during hospitalization included sertraline and intravenous fluids. Unsuccessful antibiotic therapy administered prior to Quin/Dalf therapy included vancomycin and ceftazidime. Serum sodium levels nadired below 120 mmol/L. Serum osmolarity was 268 mosm/L and urine osmolarity was 426 mosm/L. Serum sodium gradually returned to baseline (within one week) after the drug was stopped.

The authors concluded that quinupristin-dalfopristin is responsible for hyponatremia in this patient based on electrolyte changes in relation to the drug's administration. Although both small cell carcinoma and sertraline have also been associated with hyponatremia, the authors noted that changes in serum sodium were temporally associated with quinupristin-dalfopristin administration.

Cole RP et al. (Columbia Univ, New York, NY 10032) Hyponatremia associated with quinupristin-dalfopristin. Ann Intern Med 133(6):485 (Sep 19) 2000 (letter)

QUINOLONES
ALATROVAFLOXACIN
Thrombocytopenia (First Report*)

A 54-year-old inpatient developed headache and refractory epistaxis three days after starting intravenous alatrovafloxacin (300 mg) for pneumonia. Other medications included nebulized albuterol (2.5 mg), ipratropium (0.5 mg every four hours), acetaminophen (650 mg every four to six hours) and zolpidem (5 mg nightly). Platelets were decreased (7×10^3/mm^3) despite a stabilized hemoglobin and hematocrit. Despite substitution with intravenous azithromycin (500 mg daily) for alatrovafloxacin, platelet counts decreased further (2×10^3/mm^3) and petechiae were present on the oral mucous membranes. Treatment with intravenous methylprednisolone (125 mg every 12 hours) and insulin for resultant serum glucose increases were started. By discharge on hospital day eight the platelet count had increased to (60×10^3/mm^3) and was further increased on post discharge follow up six days later.

The authors concluded that is the first report of immune mediated thrombocytopenia secondary to alatrovafloxacin therapy. They recommended that clinicians should monitor patients for both liver function and bleeding during alatrovafloxacin therapy.

Gales BJ & Sulak LB (Dept Pharm, INTEGRIS Baptist Med Center, 3300 NW Expressway, Oklahoma City, OK 73112; e-mail:galesb@swosu.edu) Severe thrombocytopenia associated with alatrovafloxacin. Ann Pharmacother 34:330–334 (Mar) 2000

CIPROFLOXACIN
Bullous Pemphigoid (First Report*)

A 32-year-old patient developed blisters approximately four days after starting oral ciprofloxacin for a urinary tract infection. Other concurrent medications over the previous months included intrathecal methotrexate, granulocyte colony stimulating factor, dapsone, and itraconazole (dosages not provided). Symptoms included several erythematous bullae on the trunk and extremities but not the mouth. Histologic examination was indicative of subepidermal blistering with eosinophils. Bullous pemphigoid was verified via indirect immunofluorescence. Symptoms improved within a week after ciprofloxacin was discontinued but required treatment with oral prednisone (40 mg daily) over a four-week period. During a seven-month follow-up period the blisters did not recur and a repeat indirect immunofluorescence was negative.

The authors concluded that ciprofloxacin was responsible for bullous pemphigoid in this patient based on the temporal relationship between drug administration and the development and reversal of symptoms. No mechanism of action was provided. They cautioned clinicians to be aware of this possible cutaneous reaction when evaluating a patient with a quinolone induced cutaneous reaction.

Kimyai-Asadi A et al (Ronald O Perelman, Dept Dermatol, New York Univ Sch Med, 401 E 34th St, S-6N, NY, NY 10016; email:akimyai@yahoo.com) Ciprofloxacin induced bullous pemphigoid. J Am Acad Dermatol 42:847 (May) 2000 (letter)

CIPROFLOXACIN
Allergy

During a meningococcal infection outbreak at a university, approximately 3200 first year university students received ciprofloxacin (500 mg) as a prophylactic regimen. Of these, three students and one close contact experienced an anaphylactoid reaction. Symptoms included tight and hoarse throat, ocular and facial swelling, hypertension, pruritic rash, dyspnea, nausea, vomiting and/or cough. Treatment included intramuscular epinephrine and oral chlorpheniramine in three students with nebulized salbutamol in one. One student was hospitalized for two days. The contact individual was treated with intramuscular chlorpheniramine and hydrocortisone. One individual each had a history of asthma and penicillin allergy, respectively. Two of the three students did not have a history of atopic illness.

The authors noted that the rate of allergic response in this setting was significantly higher than incidences previously reported (1:1000 vs 1:100,000).

Burke P et al (St Bartholomew's Med Centre, Oxford OX4 1XB) Allergy associated with ciprofloxacin. Br Med J 320:679 (Mar 11) 2000 (letter)

CIPROFLOXACIN
Tendon Rupture

Two cases of tendon rupture with ciprofloxacin are reported in two adult patients after short term therapy.

Patient 1: A 38-year-old patient developed severe pain while walking approximately six months after taking a one week course of ciprofloxacin (500 mg twice daily). No other concurrent medications were provided or mentioned. Physical examination indicated complete rupture of the Achilles tendon, requiring surgical repair. Postoperative recovery was uneventful.

Patient 2: A 54-year-old patient developed marked right shoulder pain upon exertion approximately two months after starting a 10 week regimen of ciprofloxacin (500 mg twice daily) for recurrent bacterial prostatitis. The pain was unresponsive to NSAID therapy. Further examination of the area revealed a partial tear of the subscapularis tendon. Symptoms resolved within five weeks after discontinuing ciprofloxacin. Treatment included physical therapy and an unspecified NSAID regimen.

The authors suggested that these patients developed tendon rupture as a result of ciprofloxacin therapy. A possible mechanism of action included abnormal reactive healing response or cystic degeneration. The authors also cautioned clinicians to be aware of this potential complication associated with fluoroquinolone usage.

Casparian JM et al. (Univ Kansas Med Center, Div Dermatol, 4023 Wescoe, 3901 Rainbow Blvd, KC, KS 66160-7319) Quinolone and tendon rupture. S Med J 93(5): 488–491 (May) 2000

CIPROFLOXACIN AND GLYBURIDE
Interaction: Resistant Hypoglycemia

An 89-year-old nursing home resident became confused and developed slurred speech and diaphoresis approximately seven days after starting ciprofloxacin (250 mg twice daily) for acute cystitis. Chronic medications included glyburide (5 mg daily), lansoprazole (15 mg twice daily), calcitonin nasal spray (200 mcg daily), celecoxib (100 mg twice daily), docusate sodium (100 mg twice daily), senna/docusate sodium (twice daily), and citalopram (20 mg daily). Upon hospital admission, serum glucose was low (57 mg/dL) but other signs and symptoms (pulse, blood pressure, urinalysis, temperature) were within normal ranges. After ingestion of orange juice with two sugar packets, serum glucose remained low (41 mg/dL) indicating resistant hypoglycemia. Treatment included intravenous 10% dextrose and oral alimentation to maintain normal glucose levels. Serum glyburide levels were 1050 ng/mL.

The authors suggested that the addition of ciprofloxacin to this patient's stable drug regimen was responsible for the development of resistant hypoglycemia. They proposed that elevated glyburide levels were induced via ciprofloxacin inhibition of P-450 CYP3A4 isoenzymes, and suggested that close patient monitoring is warranted during combination therapy.

Roberge RJ et al (Kaplan R, Dept Emergency Med, Western Pennsylvania Hosp, 4800 Friendship Ave, Pittsburgh, PA 15224) Glyburide-ciprofloxacin interaction with resistant hypoglycemia. Ann Emerg Med 36(2):160–163 (Aug) 2000

CIPROFLOXACIN AND WARFARIN
Hypothrombinemia, Bleeding

Two patients experienced clinical bleeding due to hypothrombinemia induced by an interaction between ciprofloxacin and warfarin therapy.

Patient 1: A 50-year-old woman was admitted for lethargy, nausea, frontal headache and dysuria approximately two days after starting oral ciprofloxacin (500 mg twice daily) for a suspected urinary tract infection. Other medications upon admission included prednisone, cyclosporine, lisinopril, methotrexate, diltiazem, folate, conjugated estrogens and warfarin. One week prior to hospitalization she was stabilized on warfarin with INRs and PTs of 3.0 and 20.8, respectively. A CT of the head to investigate confusion revealed bilateral subdural hematomas. At this time, INR and PT were 8.8 and 36.5 seconds. The INR decreased to 1.0 after administration of vitamin K (10 mg). Clot evacuation was successful and the remainder of her hospital stay was uneventful. Six days post discharge, INR was within therapeutic range (2.4) on the previous warfarin dose.

Patient 2: A 56-year-old man, previously stabilized on warfarin therapy was hospitalized for refractory epistaxis approximately four days after starting oral ciprofloxacin (750 mg twice daily) for scrotal cellulitis. Upon admission, his INR and PT were 53.9 and 81.2 seconds, respectively. Other concurrent medications included amiodarone, folate, prednisone, diltiazem, lisinopril, ranitidine, furosemide, digoxin, nabumetone and methotrexate. Bleeding improved over a two day period after treatment with vitamin K (6 mg), fresh frozen plasma (12 units), nasal packing and oxymetazoline nasal spray. However, a surgical wound (post scrotal surgery) continued to bleed, requiring an additional vitamin K injection (4 mg). The INR was 1.0 on post-operative day three. INR was 2.2 on discharge while taking warfarin at previous doses.

A total of 64 similar ciprofloxacin-warfarin cases were obtained from the FDA's Spontaneous Reporting System database in April 1997. These events occurred in patients with median age of 72 yrs and bleeding problems became evident after a median of 5.5 days of ciprofloxacin therapy. The median INR and PT were 10.0 and 38.0 seconds, respectively. Sequaele was serious in 15 cases causing hospitalization, 2 cases noting bleeding and possibly responsible for one death. For the majority of cases, treatment included vitamin K alone, fresh frozen plasma alone or a combination of the two. The authors concluded that the addition of ciprofloxacin to previously stabilized warfarin therapy was responsible for bleeding in these two patients. Although an exact mechanism of action is not established, possible actions include protein binding, metabolism inhibition or interference with warfarin elimination. Clinicians were encouraged to monitor INR levels within four to five days after starting ciprofloxacin therapy.

Ellis RJ et al (Div Hematology/Oncology, Univ Kansas Med Center, 1417 Bell, 3901 Rainbow Blvd, KC, KS 66160; e-mail:rellis2@kumc.edu) Ciprofloxacin-warfarin coagulopathy: a case series. Am J Hematology 63:28–31 (Jan) 2000

LEVOFLOXACIN
QT Prolongation, Ventricular Tachycardia (First Report*)

An 88-year-old inpatient hospitalized for atrial fibrillation developed QT prolongation after starting therapy with inhaled albuterol, intravenous corticosteroids, levofloxacin (500 mg daily) and a single dose of intravenous procainamide (500 mg). By hospital days three and four the QTc intervals were increased to 464 msec and 568 msec, respectively. In addition, the patient experienced polymorphic ventricular tachycardia on hospital day four with further increases in QTc later that evening (577 msec). Levofloxacin was discontinued without other changes in medication regimens. QTc interval decreased to 437 msec within two days and no further tachycardiac episodes occurred.

The authors concluded that the appearance and resolution of symptoms was temporally related to levofloxacin administration. They also noted that this patient had underlying atrial fibrillation, which may have been a predisposition for ventricular tachycardia.

Samaha FF (Univ Pennsylvania Med Center & Philadelphia Dept of VA Med Center Philadelphia, PA) QTc interval prolongation and polymorphic ventricular tachycardia in association with levofloxacin. Am J Med 107:528–529 (Nov) 1999 (letter)

TROVAFLOXACIN
Neurotoxicity

Three case reports describe the development of neurotoxicity associated with short-term use of trovafloxacin in adult patients.

Patient 1: An 86-year-old inpatient with chronic osteomyelitis developed spontaneous muscle tremors in all extremities during intravenous trovafloxacin therapy (200 mg daily). All symptoms stopped after trovafloxacin withdrawal.

Patient 2: A 67-year-old inpatient developed tonic clonic seizures approximately 12 hours after his first trovafloxacin dose (300 mg daily). Prior antibiotic therapy included intravenous cefepime and gentamicin for two days before switching to trovafloxacin therapy. The patient was hospitalized for cellulitis and gangrene of the foot, was diabetic and had a history of seizures. Seizures did not recur after trovafloxacin was stopped.

Patient 3: A 54-year-old outpatient became confused, dizzy and developed an unsteady gait after one week of therapy with oral trovafloxacin therapy (200 mg daily). Symptoms persisted for two weeks after the completion of trovafloxacin treatment.

The authors concluded that the neurological toxicities in these patients were caused by trovafloxacin therapy and may be related to the chemical structure of the drug. They also suggested that trovafloxacin therapy should be avoided in patients with a history of seizures or neuropsychiatric disorders.

Menzies D et al (Infectious Dis Div, Winthrop-Univ Hosp, Minneola, NY) Trovafloxacin neurotoxicity. Am J Med 107(3):298–299 (Sep) 1999 (letter)

TROVAFLOXACIN
Demyelinating Polyneuropathy (First Report*)

A 50-year-old patient developed profound weakness and inability to arise from a sitting position within 36 hours after starting oral trovafloxacin (200 mg daily). Physical examination revealed proximal muscle weakness without sensory or reflex disturbances. All laboratory values were within normal limits with the exception of a slightly elevated creatinine kinase (187 U/L). Nerve conduction studies also indicated demyelinating polyneuropathy. Symptoms reversed and the patient regained strength within 72 hours after the drug was discontinued. Follow-up at six weeks revealed no further sequelae.

Based on the close temporal relationship, the authors concluded that this patient experienced polyneuropathy and muscle weakness due to trovafloxacin therapy. Although fluoroquinolones have been reported to cause weakness in patients with myasthenia gravis, this was the first case report of demyelinating polyneuropathy associated with trovafloxacin usage.

Murray CK & Wortmann GW. Trovafloxacin induced weakness due to a demyelinating polyneuropathy. S Med J 93(5):514–515 (May) 2000

TROVAFLOXACIN
Eosinophilic Hepatitis

A 66-year-old man developed nausea, vomiting, and abdominal distention approximately four weeks after starting oral trovafloxacin for a chronic sinusitis infection (100 mg daily). Other concurrent maintenance medications included losartan, metoprolol, hydrochlorothiazide, allopurinol, nabumetone, and doxepin. Physical examination revealed fever, abdominal distention and mild tachypnea. Abnormal laboratory values included elevated serum aspartate aminotransferase (537 IU/L), alanine aminotransferase (841 IU/L), alkaline phosphatase (111 IU/L) and BUN (30 mg/dL). Screenings for viral or bacterial etiologies were negative. Liver biopsy revealed a centrilobular and focal perioportal necrosis with eosinophil present. A stool sample was positive for Clostridium difficile. Treatment with prednisone and the withdrawal of trovafloxacin resulted in gradual normalization of renal and hepatic function.

The authors concluded that trovafloxacin was responsible for this patient's reversible hepatitis. A mechanism of action was not provided.

Chen HJL (Mass Gen Hosp, Boston MA 02114) Acute eosinophilic hepatitis from trovafloxacin. N Engl J Med 342(5):359–360 (Feb 3) 2000 (letter)

SULFONAMIDES
TRIMETHOPRIM/SULFAMETHOXAZOLE
Allergic Patient, Fatal Stevens Johnson Syndrome, Legal Action

A 93-year-old patient, with a known and chart documented allergy to sulfa products, was prescribed trimethoprim/sulfamethoxazole for a urinary tract infection. Despite the chart documentation, the nurse failed to check and administered the medication. Subsequently the patient developed Stevens Johnson Syndrome covering approximately 50% of the body, requiring hospitalization and eventually the cause of death. The prescriber claimed that no allergy was documented in the allergy section of the chart at the time of prescribing. A reported $1.6 million dollar settlement was reached during the trial.

Fier S vs Raju. Woman given Bactrim despite sulfa allergy—Stevens Johnson Syndrome leads to death at age 93—$1.6 million New York Settlement. Med Malpractice Verdicts, Settlements & Experts 16(4):25 (Apr) 2000

TRIMETHOPRIM-SULFAMETHOXAZOLE
Severe Hyperkalemia in Renal Transplant Patients

Two cases of severe hyperkalemia in renal transplant patients are described.

Patient 1: A 31-year-old post renal transplant patient was hospitalized for nausea, vomiting and muscle weakness approximately 10 days after starting oral trimethoprim-sulfamethoxazole (TMP/SMX: 320/1600 mg daily) at a previous hospital discharge for a recent respiratory infection. Concurrent therapy included cyclosporine A (125 mg daily), azathioprine (50 mg daily), methylprednisolone (8 mg daily), and colchicine (1.2 mg daily). Previous inpatient treatment for the respiratory infection included intravenous ceftriaxone and ofloxacin. Abnormal laboratory values noted upon admission included serum sodium (129 mmol/L), serum potassium (8.5 mmol/L), blood-urea-nitrogen (40 mg/dL), serum creatinine (3.3 mg/dL) and blood glucose (85 mg/dL). Serum cyclosporine levels were 107 ng/mL. Electrocardiac changes indicative of hyperkalemia included shortened QT interval and peaked narrow T waves. Treatment with intravenous isotonic saline, loop diuretics, methylprednisolone dose increases to 16 mg daily, and fludrocortisone acetate (0.3 mg daily) were unsuccessful in increasing the urinary excretion of potassium. Within five days after the withdrawal of TMP/SMX, serum potassium levels stabilized at 4.5 to 5.0 mmol/L. Serum potassium levels remained elevated during follow-up. During follow-up it was also discovered that the patient displayed adrenal insufficiency which may have contributed to the development of hyperkalemia.

Patient 2: A 28-year-old renal transplant patient was readmitted eight days after discharge for nausea and vomiting. Current medications included cyclosporine (125 mg daily), azathioprine (100 mg daily), methylprednisolone (48 mg daily), TMP-SMX (320/1600 mg daily), and colchicine (0.6 mg three times daily). A physical examination revealed hypotension (90/55 mmHg) and a pulse rate of 96 beats/min. Abnormal laboratory values included serum potassium (7.2 mmol/L), serum sodium (124 mmol/L), BUN (87 mg/dL) and serum creatinine (2.6 mg/dL). Electrocardiac changes indicative of hyperkalemia included shortened QT interval and peaked narrow T waves. Serum glucose level was 97 mg/dL and serum cyclosporine levels were 120 ng/mL. Within four days after the withdrawal of TMP/SMX, serum potassium levels stabilized at 4.7 mmol/L. Treatment also included intravenous isotonic saline infusion with furosemide. Urinary potassium excretion increased to 68 mmol/L.

The authors concluded that MP/SMX was a contributory factor in the development of hyperkalemia in these renal transplant patients and that such patients receiving even standard doses should be monitored for the development of this complication.

Koc M et al (Bihorac A, Univ Florida, Div Nephrology, PO Box 100224, JHMHC, Gainesville, FL 32610–0224; e-mail:azrabihorac@yahoo.com) Severe hyperkalemia in two renal transplant recipients treated with standard dose of trimethoprim-sulfamethoxazole. Am J Kidney Diseases 36(3):E18:1–6 (Sep) 2000 http://www.ajkd.org/cgi/content/abstract/36/3/E18

TETRACYCLINES
MINOCYCLINE
Chest Pain

A 42-year-old patient was hospitalized with low grade fever, cough and dyspnea within two weeks after starting minocycline therapy for chronic acne. Chest x-ray upon admission was normal. Symptoms did not progress and the patient was discharged after remaining afebrile. However, the patient was rehospitalized shortly after for significant pleuritic chest pain, which was related to inspiration and position. After extensive cardiac evaluation, no abnormalities could be located except for an atypical ECG, which indicated a coronary event. However, cardiac enzymes were not elevated and coronary angiography was within normal limits. A blood count revealed eosinophilia (13,000 × 10⁹/L). The patient was diagnosed with minocycline induced eosinophilic pericarditis. No treatment was provided, but minocycline was discontinued. Eosinophil count reversed, chest pain resolved and ECG was within normal limits at six week follow-up.

The authors concluded that minocycline induced eosinophilic pericarditis in this patient, which mimicked coronary disease. They suggested that eosinophil release may indirectly or directly stimulate the production of inflammatory mediator cytokines. They encouraged clinicians to be aware of this rare but potential complication of minocycline therapy.

Davey P & Lalloo DG (Nuffield Dept Med, John Radcliffe Hosp, Oxford OX3 9DU, UK; e-mail: patrick.davey@ndm.ox.ac.uk) Drug induced chest pain—rare but important. Postgrad Med J 76:420–422 (Jul) 2000

MINOCYCLINE
Tongue Hyperpigmentation

A 23-year-old patient developed dark spots on her tongue approximately four months after starting minocycline (100 mg twice daily) for acne vulgaris. Concurrent medication included clindamycin lotion (twice daily), and adapalene gel (nightly). Examination of the area revealed slate gray hyperpigmented patches on the dorsal and lateral portions of the tongue. However, there was no evidence of discoloration on other areas of the oral mucosa. Hyperpigmentation totally resolved within six weeks after minocycline administration was discontinued. Continued therapy with clindamycin lotion and adapalene gel was uneventful.

The authors concluded that minocycline was responsible for tongue hyperpigmentation in this patient. Several mechanisms have been proposed including the promotion of melanin and iron deposits in the epidermis. The authors recommended that although this is a rare reaction, minocycline should be considered in a differential diagnosis of localized hyperpigmentation.

Tanzi El & Hecker MS (1090 Amsterdam Ave, Ste 11B, New York, NY 10025; e-mail:pintotanzi@aol.com) Minocycline induced hyperpigmentation. Arch Fam Med 9: 687–688 (Aug) 2000 (letter)

MINOCYCLINE
Tongue Hyperpigmentation

A 23-year-old patient developed dark spots on her tongue four months after her minocycline dosage was increased from 50 mg twice daily to 100 mg twice daily. Concurrent medications included topical clindamycin applications (twice daily) and adalapene gel (nightly). The patches were slate gray and located on the tongue only. Pain and/or swelling were absent. Almost complete resolution of the patches occurred within six weeks after minocycline therapy was stopped. Clindamycin and adalapene therapies were continued without further event.

The authors concluded that minocycline was responsible for hyperpigmentation of the tongue in this patient with resolution following drug withdrawal. Although an exact mechanism is not known, the deposit of melanin may be responsible.

Tanzi EL & Hecker MS (1090 Amsterdam Ave, Suite 11B, New York, NY 10025; e-mail:pintotanzi@aol) Minocycline induced hyperpigmentation of the tongue. Arch Dermatol 136:427–428 (Mar) 2000 (letter)

TETRACYCLINE
Pseudotumor Cerebri, Vision Loss, Legal Action

A 16-year-old patient developed pseudotumor cerebri during tetracycline therapy for acne. Symptoms initially manifested as headaches, dizziness, and nausea but were not suspected to be drug related. An examination approximately 20 days later by an ophthalmologist revealed optic swelling due to elevated cranial pressure and recommended immediate treatment. A neurologist stopped the tetracycline and initiated treatment with acetazolamide to relieve elevated pressure. The patient eventually lost peripheral vision which will worsen with age. The plaintiff claimed that delay in treatment and discontinuation of drug resulted in irreversible vision loss. The defendants claimed that proper treatment was provided at all times. A $475,000 settlement was reached during arbitration sessions.

J Floyd vs Kaiser Permanente. Administration of tetracycline causes loss of vision— $475,000 California arbitration decision. Med Malpractice Verdicts, Settlements & Experts 16(8):24 (Aug) 2000

ANTINEOPLASTICS
ANTINEOPLASTICS
ANTINEOPLASTICS
ANTINEOPLASTICS
ANTINEOPLASTICS
ANTINEOPLASTICS

Drug	Interacting Drug	ADR	Page Number
Antineoplastic		Cognitive function in breast cancer patients	51
Chlorambucil		Hepatic failure*	52
Cyclophosphamide		Hepatotoxicity	53
Cyclophosphamide		CHF	53
Docetaxel		Glaucoma, fluid retention	62
Docetaxel		Cutaneous fibrosis	54
Docetaxel		Extravasation	54
Fludarabine		Hepatitis B reactivation	55
Fluorouracil	Warfarin	INR prolonged	56
Gemcitabine	Warfarin	INR prolonged	56
Interferon-alfa 2b		Pancreatitis	58
Interferon-alpha		Diabetic ketoacidosis*	57
Interferon-alpha		Delirium & autoimmune thyroiditis	57
Interferon-beta		Focal neuropathy*	59
Methotrexate		Med error, overdose (+)	60
Methotrexate		Allergic reaction (first dose)*	60
Mitoxantrone		Sinus bradycardia	61
Oxaliplatin		Hemolytic anemia^*	61
Paclitaxel		Glaucoma, fluid retention	62
Paclitaxel		Hypersensitivity reactions	62
Paclitaxel		Onycholysis	63
Tamoxifen		Endometrial cancer risk	64

* = first report
^ = death
(+) = legal action

Antineoplastics

ANTINEOPLASTIC CHEMOTHERAPY
Decreased Cognitive Function in Breast Cancer Patients

In a case control study, cognitive function was evaluated in breast cancer patients currently receiving adjuvant chemotherapy (31), in breast cancer patients who had completed adjuvant chemotherapy at least one year prior to the study (median: 2 yrs; n = 40), and in healthy control adults (36). Standard dose adjuvant chemotherapy was either oral cyclophosphamide (75 mg/m^2) on days one to 14, intravenous epirubicin (60 mg/m^2) on days one and eight, and intravenous fluorouracil (500 mg/m^2) on days one and eight. Patients received cycles every four weeks for a minimum of eight weeks (two complete cycles). A total of 16 women in the completed chemotherapy group were currently taking tamoxifen and two had previously taken tamoxifen. Patients in the control group were significantly younger than the those who currently were receiving chemotherapy and those who had completed chemotherapy (median: 41.5 yrs vs 49 yrs vs 46 yrs). Significantly more patients in both treatment groups were postmenopausal when compared to the control group (10 vs 29 vs 8, respectively). Cognitive impairment measured via the High Sensitivity Cognitive Screening Test (HSCS) revealed that there was a significant difference in the total median scores between women currently on chemotherapy compared to the control group (37 vs 26), but not compared to the women who had completed chemotherapy (34.5). This data indicated that overall cognitive function was impaired in the women currently receiving chemotherapy. In addition, a significantly higher rate of patients with moderate and severe impairment were in the current and previous chemotherapy groups when compared to controls (48.4% vs 50% vs 11.1%, respectively). When individual cognitive functions were analyzed, scores indicated that memory and language were significantly affected in the current chemotherapy group when compared to controls. In addition, there were significant differences for language and visual motor skills between the previous chemotherapy group and controls. However, there were no significant differences between the three groups in mood status, suggesting that cognitive changes were not related to mood disturbances.

The authors concluded that standard dose adjuvant chemotherapy in breast cancer patients impairs cognitive function with some residual effects after completion of therapy. The authors also noted that this data has important implications for health professionals caring for breast cancer patients, particularly for informed consent, patient counseling activities, and psychosocial support.

Brezden CB et al (Tannock IF, Dept Med Oncology, Princess Margaret Hosp, 610 University Ave, Toronto, ON M5G 2M9; e-mail:ian.tannock@uhn.on.ca) Cognitive function in breast cancer patients receiving adjuvant chemotherapy. J Clin Oncol 18(4): 2695–2701 (Jul) 2000

CHLORAMBUCIL
Acute Hepatic Failure (First Report*)

A 23-year-old patient developed nausea, vomiting, epigastric pain, anorexia, and icterus approximately three weeks after starting chlorambucil (10 mg daily) for membranous glomerulonephritis. Other chronic medications included warfarin and benazepril (no dosages provided). Elevated values included aspartate aminotransferase (2409 mU/mL), alanine aminotransferase (3303 mU/mL), total bilirubin (12.6 mg/dL), direct bilirubin (10.2 mg/dL), alkaline phosphatase (315 mU/mL), and lactate dehydrogenase (792 mU/mL). Coagulation values were also prolonged, including prothrombin time (35 seconds), INR (8.2), and partial thromboplastin time (63 seconds). Laboratory screenings for infectious and immunological etiologies were negative. Liver biopsy revealed subacute hemorrhagic necrosis with mild chronic inflammatory infiltrates in portal areas. Within three days after all medications were stopped, liver function tests began to decline. INR decreased to 2.5 by day 10. Warfarin was restarted without further event. Liver function tests normalized within six weeks after the drug discontinuation.

The authors concluded that chlorambucil was most likely responsible for hepatotoxicity in this patient as both warfarin and benazepril were administered for long periods without event. In addition, symptoms did not recur once warfarin was restarted. A possible mechanism of action included depletion of hepatocyte glutathione and increases in lipid peroxidation.

Patel SP et al (Div Nephrology & Hypertension, Harbor—UCLA Med Center, 1000 West Carson St, Box 406, Torrance CA 90509; e-mail:spatel@rei.edu) Chlorambucil induced acute hepatic failure in a patient with membranous nephropathy. Am J Kid Diseases 36(2):401–404 (Aug) 2000

CYCLOPHOSPHAMIDE (High Dose)
Congestive Heart Failure (QT Dispersion as Predictor)

The utility of corrected QT dispersion as a predictor of acute heart failure was studied in 19 consecutive patients (aged 15 to 63 yrs) scheduled to receive high dose cyclophosphamide therapy for peripheral blood stem cell transplantation. Prior to cyclophosphamide therapy all patients had received traditional chemotherapy and a baseline electrocardiogram. The chemotherapy regimen consisted of ranimustine (200 mg/m^2 for one day), cytarabine (300 mg/m^2 for four days), etoposide (300 mg/m^2 for four days), and cyclophosphamide (1400 mg/m^2 for four days). Five patients developed acute heart failure within the first eight days and had a significantly higher median baseline QT dispersion than patients who did not develop heart failure (61.6 vs 24.7 msec). Corrected QT dispersion was also higher in the heart failure group (72.5 vs 27.6 msec). In all patients who developed heart failure corrected QT dispersion was greater than 44.5 milliseconds but below 42.6 milliseconds in patients that did not develop heart failure. Median cumulative anthracycline dose was not different between the groups (161 vs 293 mg/m^2).

The authors concluded that corrected QT dispersions may be a noninvasive tool to predict the risk of acute heart failure associated with high dose cyclophosphamide therapy. They suggested that the increased QT dispersion may be indicative of local damage in the cardiac muscle, thus requiring greater ventricular recovery time. They also suggested that larger studies are needed to fully establish this relationship.

Nakamee H et al (Dept Clin Hematol, Osaka City Univ Med Sch, 1-4-3 Asahi-machi, Abeno-ku, Osaka 545-8585, Japan) QT dispersion as a predictor of acute heart failure after high dose cyclophosphamide. Lancet 355:805–806 (Mar 4) 2000 (letter)

CYCLOPHOSPHAMIDE
Hepatotoxicity

A 67-year-old patient with Sjorgen's syndrome was hospitalized for progressive jaundice. Medications included chronic low dose cyclophosphamide (50 mg every eight hours) and oral prednisolone (5 mg daily). The total estimated cumulative dose of cyclophosphamide was 40.5 grams. Although hepatomegaly was not detected, liver function tests were elevated, including alkaline phosphatase (213 U/L), SGOT (408 U/L), SGPT (269 U/L), and gamma glutamyl-transferase (430 U/L). Additional elevations were also noted in total bilirubin (506 umol/L) and direct bilirubin (366 umol/L).

Screenings for infectious etiologies were negative. Liver biopsy revealed canalicular cholestasis. Liver function normalized within six weeks after cyclophosphamide was discontinued.

The authors suggested that continuous low dose cyclophosphamide was related to liver damage in this patient and suggested that liver function monitoring should be regularly performed in patients receiving the drug.

Mok CC et al (Div Rheumatology, Div Hepatology, Dept Med, Queen Mary Hosp, Pokfulam, Hong Kong) Cumulative hepatotoxicity induced by continuous low-dose cyclophosphamide therapy. Am J Gastroenterol 95(3):845–846 (Mar) 2000

DOCETAXEL
Cutaneous Fibrosis

A 38-year-old patient with recurrent metastatic breast cancer developed progressive incoordination and weakness accompanied by a cutaneous sclerosis on the lower extremities, lower trunk and distal upper extremities (involving approximately 50% of body surface). These changes occurred after approximately 18 months of cyclic docetaxel therapy (125 mg/m^2 every four weeks) and were preceded by dependent leg edema. Concurrent therapy included dexamethasone as premedication, anastrazole (dosage not provided), and local brain radiation treatment. Although neurological testing was within normal limits, it was suggested that strength deficits were related to the mild to moderate fibrosis found during skin biopsy. Other findings also included perivascular inflammatory infiltrates between the epidermis and adipose layers. Normal laboratory values included but were not limited to complete blood count, other chemistry profiles, sedimentation rates, antinuclear antibodies and creatinine phosphokinase. Post docetaxel discontinuation, cutaneous tissues softened within three weeks with almost complete resolution and no functional impairment at six weeks.

The authors noted that this is only the second report and fourth patient to develop cutaneous fibrosis during cyclic docetaxel therapy. Although an exact mechanism was not proposed, several possible pathways were suggested, including increased fibroblast activation leading to increased collagen deposition and changes in vascularity of the skin.

Cleveland MG et al (Div Dermatology, Burlington Med Center, 610 N 4th St, Suite 4B, Burlington, IA, 52601) Cutaneous fibrosis induced by docetaxel: A case report. Cancer 68:1078–1081 (Mar 1) 2000

DOCETAXEL
Extravasation, Tissue Injury

A 71-year-old patient developed an infiltration in the left hand after approximately 100 mL of a docetaxel infusion was infused (0.48 mg/mL).

Initially there were no symptoms in the hand and the infusion was restarted in the right hand. However, six days after the extravasation, the skin on the left hand became erythematous which progressed to severe edema and pain over the next 24 hours, despite treatment with a hot-pack. Treatment with oral cephalexin (500 mg four times daily) for 10 days did not alleviate symptoms. Repeated examination on day four of antibiotic therapy revealed a grade 4 local skin reaction. Antibiotic therapy was continued along with NSAIDs and mild opioids for pain. Increased blistering covered the entire dorsum of the left hand with subsequent desquamation. Full recovery of hand function returned over the next four weeks with physical therapy.

The authors noted that this is the first reported case of significant tissue injury and desquamation with docetaxel extravasation during drug administration. The authors suggested that docetaxel, like other taxanes, may share similar vesicant activities.

Raley J et al (Div Gyn Oncol, Dept Ob/Gyn, Univ Iowa Hosp & Clinics, Iowa City, IA 52242) Docetaxel extravasation causing significant delayed tissue injury. Gynecologic Oncology 78:259–260 (Aug) 2000

FLUDARABINE
Hepatitis B Reactivation

Two patients with HBs Ag-positive chronic lymphocytic leukemia developed subacute and chronic hepatic injury during fludarabine chemotherapy.

Patient 1: A 57-year-old patient with stage IV chronic lymphocytic leukemia developed hepatitis B virus reactivations during two courses of fludarabine/cyclophosphamide chemotherapy (dosages not provided). The initial reactivation resulted in hepatitis B virus DNA titers of 843 pg/mL, but spontaneously resolved within two months. The second reactivation resulted in hepatitis B virus DNA titers of 2,000 pg/mL and required treatment with famcyclovir (1.5 grams/day). Liver biopsy revealed portal fibrotic expansion and fibrosis. Platelet counts returned to baseline after 10 days of therapy and hepatitis B virus DNA titers decreased to 58 pg/mL. Within one month, all laboratory screenings were within normal limits and hepatitis B virus DNA titers were negative. The patient was able to proceed with scheduled chemotherapy courses.

Patient 2: A 59-year-old patient with stage II chronic lymphocytic leukemia developed ascites and splenomegaly after five courses of fludarabine chemotherapy (dosages not provided). Hepatitis B virus DNA titers were elevated (950 pg/mL) and indicative of a hepatitis B virus reactivation. Treatment with famicyclovir (1.5 grams daily) for one month was not successful in reducing hepatitis B virus DNA titers (4500 pg/mL), requiring substitution with lamuvidine (300 mg daily).

The authors concluded that fludarabine therapy in these two patients was responsible for hepatitis B reactivation. One of the proposed mechanisms is that fludarabine exacerbates the immune deficiency of chronic lymphocytic leukemia, permitting increased hepatitis B virus replication. They suggested close monitoring of chronic lymphocytic leukemia patients taking fludarabine based chemotherapy.

Yagci M et al (No site provided) Fludarabine and risk of hepatitis B virus reactivation in chronic lymphocytic leukemia. Am J Hematol 64(3):233–234 (Jul) 2000

FLUOROURACIL AND WARFARIN
Interaction: Increased Anticoagulation

In a retrospective hospital review over a three year period, five cancer patients who received concurrent warfarin and 5-fluorouracil (5-FU) were identified to examine the possibility of a drug interaction. Prior to chemotherapy, all patients were stabilized on warfarin therapy (INRs: 2-3) and monitored monthly via an anticoagulation clinic. However, after chemotherapy started, patients required a mean reduction of 44% in warfarin dosing to maintain target INRs. In four patients who received full 5–FU doses, warfarin dosage reductions were 50%. The mean warfarin dose prior to and during chemotherapy was 40.66 mg and 24 mg, respectively. Two patients required hospitalization, one for major retroperitoneal bleeding and the other for the administration of fresh frozen plasma.

The authors suggested that this data is indicative of a clinically significant interaction between 5-FU and warfarin and that further prospective controlled trials are needed to determine definitive causality.

Kolesar JM et al (Sch Pharmacy, Univ Wisconsin—Madison, 425 North Charter St, Madison, WI 53706-1515) Warfarin-5FU interaction—a consecutive case series. Pharmacotherapy 19(12):1445–1449 (Dec) 1999

GEMCITABINE AND WARFARIN
Interaction: Increased INRs

A 63-year-old man, previously stabilized on warfarin therapy (57.5 mg weekly), experienced increased INRs (3.52 from 1.94) after receiving the first dose of gemcitabine (2380 mg per week over 30 minutes for three weeks). Other concurrent medications included potassium chloride, digoxin, isosorbide dinitrate, simvastatin, ranitidine, multivitamins, furosemide and diltiazem. During a two-week rest period between gemcitabine cycles, INRs returned to therapeutic range (2.08 to 2.13) once the warfarin dose was reduced (52.5 mg weekly). However, the INR increased again to 3.58 after the second gemcitabine cycle was started, requiring a further reduction in warfarin dosage (50 mg weekly). INRs became subtherapeutic after gemcitabine was discontinued and warfarin doses were gradually increased. Periodic liver function monitoring revealed elevations during chemotherapy cycles.

The authors concluded that decreased warfarin doses were needed because of gemcitabine-induced hepatotoxicity, possibly decreasing warfarin metabolism or synthesis of clotting factors.

Kinikar SA & Kolsear JM (Univ Wisconsin-Madison Sch Pharmacy, 425 North Charter St, Madison, WI 53706–1515) Identification of a gemcitabine-warfarin interaction. Pharmacotherapy 19(11):1331–1333 (Nov) 1999

INTERFERON ALPHA
Severe Diabetic Ketoacidosis (First Report*)

A 39-year-old diabetic patient hospitalized for chronic hepatitis C received intravenous interferon-beta (6×10^6 units/day) as therapy. At the time of admission, chronic insulin doses were 22 units daily for 13 years. During hospitalization, however, glucose control deteriorated requiring larger doses of insulin (50 units daily) to maintain normoglycemic control. Hemoglobin A1C was 11.5%. After four weeks of therapy, intramuscular interferon-alpha was substituted (10×10^6 units/day). After approximately three days of therapy, the patient became confused, hypotensive with severe arrhythmias, requiring transfer to an intensive care unit. Abnormal laboratory values indicated diabetic ketoacidosis with shock, including pH (6.832), HCO3 (2.2 mmol/L), hemoglobin A1C (14.3%), blood glucose (76.8 mmol/L), and total ketone body (14,320 mmol/L). Screenings for infectious etiologies were negative. Therapy included insulin, mechanical ventilation, continuous hemodiafiltration and hemodynamic support. Recovery was progressive with eventual ICU discharge after five days.

The authors noted that this was the first case report of interferon related diabetic ketoacidosis. They also suggested that interferon alpha has a stronger effect on glucose control than interferon beta. However, an exact mechanism of action was not provided. This publication did not indicate if the suspected product was interferon-alpha 2a or alpha 2b.

Hayakawa M et al (Dept Anesthesiology & Critical Care Med, Hokkaido Univ Sch Med, N17 W5, Kita-ku, Sapporo 060-8648, Japan) Development of severe diabetic ketoacidosis with shock after changing interferon-beta into interferon-alpha for chronic hepatitis C. Intensive Care Med 26:1008 (Jul) 2000 (letter)

INTERFERON-ALPHA
Delirium with Autoimmune Thyroiditis

A 23-year-old patient developed delirium, requiring hospitalization, 10 days after the cessation of a six month regimen of interferon for a right nephrectomy for renal cell carcinoma. A brain CT scan was negative for metastases. Abnormal laboratory values included TSH (53.97 microU/mL), free triodothyronine (2.24 pg/mL), and free thyroxine (3.6 pg/mL). Thyroid replacement, started on hospital day seven, resulted in gradual symptom improvement without the use of neuroleptics. Thyroid function returned to normal within three weeks. The patient was amnesiac for the first 10 hospital days.

The authors concluded that delirium was caused by interferon induced thyroid disorder.

Nibuya M et al. (Tochgi, Japan) Delirium with autoimmune thyroiditis induced by interferon alpha. Am J Psychiatry 157(10):1705–1706 (Oct) 2000 (letter)

INTERFERON ALFA-2b
Acute Pancreatitis

Two cases of acute pancreatitis were reported in patients shortly after receiving treatment with interferon alfa-2b for chronic hepatitis C.

Patient 1: A 40-year-old patient was hospitalized with abdominal pain, nausea, and vomiting of approximately 12 weeks duration. Fifteen weeks earlier he started treatment with subcutaneous interferon alfa 2b (three times weekly) and oral ribavirin (1200 mg daily) for chronic hepatitis C. Other concurrent medications included omeprazole (40 mg daily) and mebeverine (400 mg daily). Abdominal tenderness was apparent upon physical examination. Both oral ribavirin and subcutaneous interferon were discontinued. Elevated laboratory values also included gamma-glutamyl transferase (124 U/L), serum amylase (136 U/L), serum lipase (740 U/L), and C-reactive protein (30.9 mg/L). Other laboratory values were within normal ranges. Within five days the symptoms had resolved and lipase and amylase levels had normalized. However, within hours after rechallenge with interferon-alfa-2b, abdominal pain recurred and serum lipase increased to 348 U/L. Although relapse of acute pancreatitis was partially attributed to initiation of solid food, interferon was stopped again. Serum lipase returned to baseline within four days. Rechallenge with interferon-alfa-2b once more also resulted in elevations of serum lipase (1903 U/L) without clinical symptoms. Interferon therapy was not restarted and the patient remained asymptomatic during a one year follow-up period.

Patient 2: A 38-year-old was hospitalized with abdominal pain and nausea. Medications included intracavernous papaverine injected two hours prior to admission and an initial subcutaneous dose of interferon-alfa-2b (5 million units). Abdominal pain and tenderness was apparent upon physical examination. Elevated laboratory values upon admission included serum amylase (137 U/L), serum lipase (1014 U/L), aspartate aminotransferase

(31 U/L), and alanine aminotransferase (69 U/L). Levels of other laboratory measures were within normal ranges. Amylase and lipase levels normalized within two days after the drugs were discontinued. However, serum amylase and lipase levels increased again when interferon was restarted (3 million units) five weeks later. Despite increased levels (123 U/L and 456 U/L, respectively), treatment was continued. Severe abdominal pain also recurred two weeks later. At this time serum lipase and amylase levels were within normal ranges and CT scans revealed no abnormalities of the gall bladder, bile ducts or pancreas. Treatment was discontinued and the patient remained asymptomatic during a two-year follow-up period. Intracavernous papaverine was continued without event.

The authors concluded that interferon was responsible for acute pancreatitis in both patients. A mechanism of action was not proposed but the authors noted that both patients had serum triglycerides within normal limits, and thus, pancreatic changes were not related to triglyceride changes. They cautioned clinicians to consider interferon-alfa-2b as a potential cause of acute pancreatitis.

Eland IA et al (Stricker BHC, Erasmus Med Center, Rotterdam, Dijkzigt, Lab of Internal Med II, PO Box 2040, 3000 CA, L448, Rotterdam, The Netherlands; e-mail:inw2.azr.nl) Acute pancreatitis attributed to the use of interferon alfa-2b. Gastronenterology 119: 230–233 (Jul) 2000

INTERFERON—BETA
Focal Neuropathy (First Report*)

A 39-year-old multiple sclerosis patient developed a painful, livedoid pattern on the posterior aspect of the upper arm at an injection site used for interferon-beta 1b over the previous three years. Symptoms progessed to a necrotic ulcer, accompanied by tingling in the dorsal aspect of the thumb. No motor or reflex abnormalities were observed. Although the livedo and ulcer resolved over a one month period, the tingling sensation persisted for 10 months before it resolved. Other etiologies were dismissed due to negative lab screenings. Neurophysiological testing, performed three months after onset of the problem, indicated radial neuropathy via an 80% reduction in the compound muscle action potential amplitude in the right radial nerve near the injection site. This conduction block also resolved after 10 months.

The authors suggested that in this patient, conduction block may have occurred via ischemic local damage induced by interferon injections. They also recommended that certain injection sites should be avoided to preserve effects on nearby peripheral nerves, including the posterior aspect of the arm (radial nerve), the lateral abdominal wall and anterior superior iliac spine (lateral demoral cutaneous nerve), and the upper aspects of the buttocks (sciatic nerve).

Creange A & Lefaucheur JP (Serv Neurologie, Centre Hospitalier, Univ Henri Mondor, 94010 Creteol Cedex, Fance; e-mail:creange@univ.paris12.fr) Focal neuropathy associated with cutaneous necrosis at the site of interferon beta injection for multiple sclerosis. J Neurol Neurosurg Psychiatry 68:388 (Mar) 2000 (letter)

METHOTREXATE
First Dose Allergic Reaction (First Report*)

A 16-year-old patient with widespread metastatic disease developed an urticarial rash on his trunk and lower extremities within 30 minutes after receiving the first dose of high dose methotrexate (12 gm/m^2 for four hours weekly). Prior to administration, 5% glucose and ondansetron were also administered for the first time. Treatment with intravenous diphenhydramine (0.5 mg/kg) resulted in rapid disappearance of the rash within 20 minutes. Readministration of methotrexate was uneventful and no other symptoms of an allergic reaction were observed.

The authors concluded that the patient's metastatic disease might have possibly contributed to this reaction. Antibody synthesis initially directed against other antigenic determinants may have caused a subsequent cross-reaction to methotrexate. They noted that this was the first report of an allergic reaction after the first infusion of methotrexate.

Postovsky S et al (Arush WB, Dept Pediatric Hemato-Oncology, Rambam Med Center, POB 9602, Haifa 31096, Israel; e-mail:m_benarush@rambam.health.gov.il) Allergic reaction to high-dose methotrexate. Med & Pediatric Oncol 35:131–132 (Sep) 2000

METHOTREXATE
Overdose, Medication Error, Legal Action

A 77-year-old inpatient inadvertently received much higher doses of methotrexate (2.5 mg three times daily) as a result of an incorrectly written order. Typical dosing prior to hospitalization was three 2.5 mg tablets on Saturdays only for rheumatoid arthritis. The dosing error was recognized by the pharmacy and dosing was corrected. However, four days after a post surgical repair for an abdominal aortic aneurysm, methotrexate was incorrectly prescribed again and administered at this dosage for three days. Although methotrexate administration was stopped, the antidote was not administered for almost four days after the last methotrexate dose. In addition, it was administered orally rather than parenterally. Bone marrow toxicity ensued, resulting in prolonged hospitalization until the patient's death. A $645,000 settlement was reached.

Co-administrators of the Estate of HC Richards vs USA. Overdose of methotrexate given at VA hospital—proper antidote not given and antidote given too late—death a year later—$645,000 Tennessee settlement. Med Malpractice Verdicts, Settlements & Experts 16(6):20 (Jun) 2000

MITOXANTRONE
Sinus Bradycardia

A 73-year-old inpatient with acute myelogenous leukemia developed asymptomatic sinus bradycardia (30 to 40 beats/minute) on day two of mitoxantrone therapy (dosage not provided). Prechemotherapy electrocardiograms were within normal ranges. Other medications were not mentioned in the case report. Heart rate returned to baseline within six days after mitoxantrone infusion was completed. The remainder of the hospital stay was uneventful resulting in eventual discharge. No complications were noted during a follow-up period of three months.

The authors noted that this is only the third published case report of mitoxantrone induced bradycardia. They also encouraged clinicians to be aware of this possible side effect. No mechanism of action was provided.

Chan-Tack K (305 Nikki Way, Columbia, MO 65203) Sinus bradycardia due to mitoxantrone. South Med J 93(4):440 (Apr) 2000 (letter)

OXALIPLATIN
Fatal Hemolytic Anemia (First Report*)

A 66-year-old woman with metastatic colorectal adenocarcinoma developed severe lower back pain, fever and chills during an oxaliplatin infusion. She had previously received 44 chemotherapy cycles, which consisted of oxaliplatin (100 mg/m^2), folinic acid (200 mg/m^2), 5-fluorouracil bolus (400 mg/m^2) for two days every two weeks. Despite stopping the chemotherapy, she developed scleral icterus and dark urine. Corticosteroid therapy was initiated (no dosages provided) but was not successful in relieving symptoms. Abnormal laboratory values included decreased hemoglobin (48 g/L), elevated bilirubin (470 umol/L), elevated LDH (8505 IU/L), and elevated creatinine (471 umol/L). Despite intensive care support treatment, multiple blood transfusions (23 units of packed red cells), corticosteroids and dialysis, the patient expired. Blood samples revealed that oxaliplatin serum concentrations were 331.5 mg/L with a hemolysis titer of 1/1 and agglutination titer of 1/256.

The authors noted that this is the first published report of hemolytic anemia with oxaliplatin. No mechanism of action was provided.

Desrame J et al (Serv de Pathol Digestive, Hopital d'Instruction des Amees Begin, 69 Ave de Paris, 94163 Saint Mande Cedex, France; e-mail:capgastr@club-internet.fr) Oxaliplatin induced haemolytic anaemia. Lancet 354:1179–1180 (Oct 2) 1999

PACLITAXEL, DOCETAXEL
Glaucoma, Fluid Retention

A 31-year-old woman with metastatic breast cancer developed fluid retention after the first cycle and vision loss after the fifth cycle of chemotherapy. Cycles consisted of docetaxel infusion (100 mg/m^2) every 21 days preceded by prednisolone (50 mg) at 12 and three hours prior to the dose. Although an ophthalmologic examination revealed a significant increase in intraocular pressure (44 mmHg in both eyes) the fundus and visual field examinations were normal. A gonioscopic evaluation revealed a wide open angle consistent with open-angle glaucoma. Intraocular pressure gradually decreased after docetaxel was discontinued and ophthalmic betaxolol was initiated. Months later she was restarted on paclitaxel cycles (135 mg/m^2) preceded by methylprednisolone (130 mg) 12 and six hours prior to dosing. Fluid retention recurred after two cycles and open-angle glaucoma recurred after three cycles (35 and 40 mm Hg). Despite treatment with oral acetazolamide (no dosage provided) and ocular betaxolol and latanoprost, intraocular pressures did not improve during continued chemotherapy. However, chemotherapy was stopped shortly after due to changes noted in fundoscopy.

The authors noted that glaucoma occurred after the development of fluid retention in this patient, which may have precipitated the increased ocular pressures. Although an exact mechanism of action was not provided the authors concluded that the taxene drugs were responsible for these ocular effects.

Fabre-Guillevin E et al (Dr Allen Ravaud, Dept Med, Instit Bergonie, Reg Cancer Center, 180 Rue de Saint-Genes, 33076, Bordeaux Cedex, France; e-mail:ravaud @bergonie.org) Taxene induced glaucoma. Lancet 354:1181–1182 (Oct 2) 1999 (letter)

PACLITAXEL
Hypersensitivity Reactions Related to Bee Sting Allergies

In a retrospective case control chart review, 19 patients with a documented anaphylaxis after paclitaxel administration were compared to 38 controls and examined for allergy history. When compared to control patients, a significantly higher percentage of paclitaxel—sensitive patients were allergic to bee stings (0% vs 36.8%) and animals (0% vs 15.7%). There were no differences between the groups for plant, drug or all allergies. The mean paclitaxel dose prior to anaphylaxis was 4.26 mg and pretreatment included dexamethasone, diphenhydramine and cimetidine. Approximately one-third of the patients were able to continue therapy after receiving 24 hours of intravenous steroid dosing.

The authors suggested that all patients should be questioned about their allergy history prior to paclitaxel administration and that patients with allergy history, particularly bee stings, should receive oral dexamethasone premedication.

Grosen E et al (Dept Ob/Gyn, Univ Wisconsin Hosp & Clin, 600 Highland Ave, H4/636 CSC, Madison, WI 53792) Paclitaxel hypersensitivity reactions related to bee stings. Lancet 354:288–289 (Jan 22) 2000 (letter)

PACLITAXEL
Onycholysis

In a prospective evaluation of 178 cancer patients receiving either paclitaxel (91) or doxorubicin (187), onycholysis occurred in five of 21 patients receiving greater than six week cycles of paclitaxel. None of the patients receiving doxorubicin developed onycholysis. Five case reports are described.

Patient 1: A 55-year-old patient with metastatic breast cancer developed onycholysis of all the fingernails after completing 12 courses of paclitaxel therapy (100 mg/m^2). The toenails were not evaluated. After metastatic disease recurred, paclitaxel was discontinued. Progression of onycholysis was not determined due to loss of follow-up.

Patient 2: A 71-year-old patient with pulmonary cancer and spinal metastasis developed onycholysis of all toe and fingernails after completing 14 courses of weekly paclitaxel therapy (100 mg/m^2). All nails were lost and skin of the fingertip was inflamed. After treatment was discontinued, normal nail growth recurred. Once paclitaxel therapy was restarted, the patient protected the nails from sunlight and onycholysis did not recur.

Patient 3: A 45-year-old breast cancer patient developed onycholysis after completing 15 courses of weekly paclitaxel therapy (100 mg/m^2). Painless separation of most fingernails and one toenail was accompanied by mild inflammation of the fingertip skin. Onycholysis resolved with protection from sunlight, despite continued paclitaxel administration.

Patient 4: A 44-year-breast cancer patient with bone metastases developed onycholysis of multiple fingernails after completing 18 courses of paclitaxel therapy (100 mg/m^2 weekly then biweekly). No fingertip skin inflammation was observed. Onycholysis resolved with nail protection from sunlight, despite continued paclitaxel administration.

Patient 5: A 70-year-old breast cancer patient with bone metastases developed onycholysis and leukonychia after receiving her 14th dose of paclitaxel (100 mg/m^2). All fingernails were involved but no toenails. Onycholysis resolved with nail protection from sunlight, despite continued paclitaxel administration.

The authors concluded that paclitaxel was responsible for onycholysis in these patients, possibly precipitated by sunlight exposure. All of the cases reported occurred in the late spring and summertime when sunlight exposure is more common. The authors suggested nail protection from sunlight (via gloves or artificial nails) in patients receiving paclitaxel.

Hussain S et al (Braverman AS, Box 55, Health Science Center at Brooklyn, State Univ of New York, 450 Clarkson Ave, Brooklyn, NY 11203-2098) Onycholysis as a complication of systemic chemotherapy. Report of five cases associated with prolonged weekly paclitaxel therapy and review of the literature. Cancer 88:2367–2371 (May 15) 2000

TAMOXIFEN
Risk of Endometrial Cancer

In a nationwide case control study, 299 cases of confirmed endometrial cancer at least three months after breast cancer diagnosis were identified and compared to 860 controls with breast cancer only. Approximately 36.1% and 28.5% of the case and controls, respectively were currently receiving or had taken tamoxifen therapy. The median duration of therapy was longer in the case group (24 vs 18 months). The median time between diagnosis of breast and endometrial cancer was 40 months (range: 4 to 235 months). The unadjusted relative risk associated with tamoxifen use was 1.5. However, risks were increased with longer tamoxifen use. The adjusted relative risk for endometrial cancer associated with less than two years of therapy was 1.0, was 1.9 for two to five years of therapy, and was 6.6 for five or more years. Daily dose did not affect the risk of endometrial cancer when total duration of use was examined. Factors which also significantly increased the risk of endometrial cancer included weight, body mass index, hormone replacement therapy, and other hormonal therapy. A total of 21 case patients died due to endometrial cancer during a median follow-up of 30 months. The three year survival rate for endometrial cancer was significantly worse for long term tamoxifen users (76% for users > five years) as compared to either users for two to five years (85%) or nonusers (94%).

The authors concluded that long-term tamoxifen users were at greater risk of endometrial cancer than non-users. However, they also stated that the significant therapeutic benefit of the drug on breast cancer survival rates outweighed the increased mortality from endometrial cancer.

Bergman L et al (van Leeuwen FE: Dept Epidemiology, Netherlands Cancer Instit, 1066 CX Amsterdam, Netherlands; e-mail: fvleeuw@nki.nl) Risk and prognosis of endometrial cancer after tamoxifen for breast cancer. Lancet 356:881–887 (Sep 9) 2000

BLOOD

BLOOD

BLOOD

BLOOD

BLOOD

BLOOD

Drug	Interacting Drug	ADR	Page Number
Abciximab		Thrombocytopenia	67
Alteplase		Anaphylactic reactions	68
Clopidogrel		Acute arthritis	69
Clopidogrel		Ageusia	69
Clopidogrel		Hemolytic uremic syndrome*	70, 71
Clopidogrel		Thrombotic thrombocytopenia	71
Dalteparin		Alopecia*	72
Epoetin		Cerebral venous thrombosis	73
Epoetin		Pyrogenic reactions	73
Ferrous sulfate		Hemosidersosis	74
Heparin		Thrombocytopenia (+)	74, 75
Streptokinase		Hypersensitivity, Off-label use	75
Ticlodipine		Aplastic anemia	75
Warfarin		Hemorrhage mimics pelvic tumor*	76
Warfarin	Celecoxib	Coagulation changes	76
Warfarin	Ciprofloxacin	Hypothrombinemia, bleeding	77
Warfarin	Fluorouracil	INR prolonged	78
Warfarin	Gemcitabine	INR prolonged	79
Warfarin	Methylsalicylate	Anticoagulation potentiation	79
Warfarin	Miconazole (vaginal)	INR increased*	80
Warfarin	Nabumetone	INR increased*	81
Warfarin	Tolterodine	INR prolonged	81

* = first report
^ = death
(+) = legal action

Blood

ABCIXIMAB WITH CLOPIDOGREL OR TICLOPIDINE
Incidence of Thrombocytopenia

The incidence of thrombocytopenia was assessed in a retrospective review of 174 consecutive patients undergoing coronary stent implementation with administration of abciximab and either ticlopidine or clopidogrel. Sixteen of the patients (9.2%) developed thrombocytopenia with four (2.3%) cases rated as severe. Reaction onset was less than 24 hours in all but one patient. Patients who had received clopidogrel loading dose (300 mg) with abciximab had a higher rate than with abciximab alone (24% vs 2.5% to 5.2%).

The authors concluded that the combination of a 300 mg loading clopidogrel dose with abciximab is associated with a significantly higher incidence of thrombocytopenia.

Dillon WC et al. (Ritchies ME, Krannert Instit of Cardiol, Indiana Univ, 1111 W 10th St, Indianapolis, Indiana 46202; e-mail:miritchi@iupui.edu) Incidence of thrombocytopenia following coronary stent replacement using abciximab plus clopidogrel or ticlopidine. Cathet Cardiovasc Intervent 50:426–430 (Sep) 2000

ABCIXIMAB
Thrombocytopenia

A 64-year-old inpatient developed shivering and transient hypotension within the first hour after receiving abciximab bolus (25 mg) and infusion (8 mg/hr for 12 hrs). The infusion was stopped for one hour and restarted. After eight hours, the platelet count was decreased (17×10^9/L). Despite discontinuation of the infusion, the platelet count continued to decrease (1×10^9/L), requiring 10 units of platelets. The preoperative platelet count was 209×10^9/L, indicating that drug administration was responsible. An abdominal scan performed because of abdominal pain revealed a mild to moderate retroperitoneal hematoma. The patient also experienced hematuria. An additional 10 units of platelets were administered with a subsequent increase in the platelet count to 150×10^9/L. Further recovery was uneventful.

The authors concluded that abciximab was responsible for the development of thrombocytopenia in this patient. Despite a full recovery in this patient with only minor effects, the authors recommend routine measurement of platelets four hours after abciximab administration.

Butler R & Hubner PJB (Dept Cardiology, Glenfield Hosp, Groby Rd, Leicester LE3 9QP, UK) Acute severe thrombocytopenia after treatment with ReoPro (abciximab). Heart 83:e5–e6 (Apr) 2000 (http://www.heartjnl.com/cgi/con-tent/ fill/83/4/e5)

ALTEPLASE
Anaphylactoid Reactions, Angioedema

Reports of anaphylactoid reactions are described in two patients during alteplase treatment for acute ischemic stroke.

Patient 1: A 74-year-old woman developed an urticarial rash approximately 45 minutes after an alteplase bolus and infusion (0.9 mg/kg) was started for suspected acute ischemic stroke. The infusion was immediately discontinued (38 mg received). Other concurrent medications prior to admission included aspirin, losartan, furosemide, diltiazem, digoxin, atorvastatin, acarbose, glyburide, and a nitroglycerin transdermal patch. Despite prompt discontinuation of the alteplase, symptoms progressed to include swelling of the tongue and periorbital areas, and significant hypotension (90/40 mmHg). Treatment with intravenous hydrocortisone (100 mg), ranitidine (50 mg) and diphenhydramine (50 mg) did not immediately reverse symptoms, which worsened, requiring intubation. The patient was eventually admitted to the intensive care unit for oropharyngeal hemorrhage related to the intubation and small midline brainstem hemorrhage. Two weeks after hospitalization the patient died after developing ventricular arrhythmias. Autopsy was not performed but the family indicated that the patient had experienced eight angioedema episodes within the prior 14 years.

Patient 2: A 76-year-old woman developed angioedema symptoms within 30 minutes after receiving an alteplase infusion (0.9 mg/kg) for suspected ischemic stroke. Rash or hypotension did not occur. The only other concurrent medication upon admission was an ACE inhibitor (specific product not provided). After treatment with intravenous methylprednisolone (80 mg), diphenhydramine (50 mg), and ranitidine (25 mg), symptoms resolved over the next several hours.

The authors noted that angioedema has been reported with the use of alteplase in the treatment of myocardial infarction but not commonly with the use of this drug for therapy of ischemic stroke. They concluded that these two cases were anaphylactoid reactions related to intravenous alteplase infusions. A possible suggested mechanism of action included activation of the complement and kinin cascades by alteplase. They also noted that the first patient may have had an undiagnosed C1 esterase inhibitor deficiency resulting in an exaggerated complement cascade reaction and severe oropharyngeal angioedema. They noted that the second patient was also taking an ACE inhibitor, which may have predisposed the patient to this type of reaction.

Hill MD et al. (Dept Clin Neurosciences, Univ Calgary, MRG 005, Foothills Hosp, 1403 29th St NW, Calgary AB T2N 2T9; e-mail:michael.hill@crha-health.ab.ca) Anaphylactoid reactions and angioedema during alteplase treatment of acute ischemic stroke. Can Med Assoc J 162(9):1281–1284 (May 2) 2000

CLOPIDOGREL
Acute Arthritis

Two cases of acute arthritis and tendonitis during clopidogrel use in elderly patients are described.

Patient 1: A 76-year-old patient developed extensive pruritis (without rash) and painful swelling of the finger joints approximately two weeks after starting clopidogrel (75 mg once daily). Concurrent medications included diltiazem (120 mg twice daily) and aspirin (150 mg once daily). Elevated laboratory values included erythrocyte sedimentation rate (86 mm/h) and C-reactive protein (81 mg/L). Serum urate concentrations, however, were within normal ranges and did not indicate acute gout mechanisms. One week after clopidogrel was stopped, the symptoms improved.

Patient 2: A 63-year-old patient sought medical attention for severe pain in the right knee, approximately three weeks after starting clopidogrel (75 mg once daily). Concurrent medications included only lisinopril (20 mg once daily). Although serum urate concentrations were within normal ranges, the erythrocyte sedimentation rate was elevated (47 mm/h). Symptoms resolved after clopidogrel discontinuation, but a specific time period of recovery was not provided.

The authors noted that these cases represented the second and third reports of arthritis potentially linked with clopidogrel therapy. A mechanism of action was not discussed.

Garg A et al (Dept Cardiology, Royal Bournemouth Hosp, Bournemouth Dorset BH8 8DH) Br Med J 20:483 (Feb 19) 2000 (letter)

CLOPIDOGREL
Ageusia

Two patients who developed reversible ageusia while taking clopidogrel therapy are described.

Patient 1: A 76-year-old patient developed loss of taste within six weeks after she was switched to clopidogrel (75 mg daily) from aspirin therapy due to gastrointestinal intolerance. The sense of smell was not altered and routine laboratory tests with a cranial scan were within normal limits. Ageusia partially reversed within 20 days after clopidogrel therapy was stopped. Full recovery of taste was experienced several days later.

Patient 2: A 64-year-old patient developed ageusia within two months after starting clopidogrel therapy (75 mg daily) for transient cerebral ischemia. Previous therapy included aspirin (300 mg daily). The sense of smell was not altered. Within six weeks after clopidogrel was discontinued and aspirin therapy was substituted, full recovery of taste resumed. However, taste loss recurred within two weeks after clopidogrel therapy with a different commercial preparation was restarted for a recent transient cerebral ischemic attack. Recovery recurred within six weeks after the drug was stopped.

The authors noted that these were the first published reports of reversible ageusia with clopidogrel. A mechanism of action was not established.

Golka K et al (Instit Occupational Physiology, Univ Dortmund, Ardeystrasse 67, 44139 Dortmund) Reversible ageusia as an effect of clopidogrel treatment. Lancet 355:465–466 (Feb 5) 2000 (letter)

CLOPIDOGREL
Hemolytic Uremic Syndrome (First Report*)

A 54-year-old man developed fatigue, diffuse petechaie, hematuria and rash over lower extremities approximately two weeks after starting clopidogrel (75 mg daily) post coronary stenting. Other concurrent medications included aspirin, metoprolol, ranitidine, and terazosin. A 24-hour abciximab infusion was administered immediately post stenting. Although a physical examination was unremarkable with the exception of the rash, laboratory tests revealed an increased urea nitrogen (40 mg/dL) and creatinine (2.0 mg/dL). Lactate dehydrogenase was 933 /L and total bilirubin concentration (3.0 mg/dL). Blood counts included hematocrit (36%), white blood cell (9.1 × 10^9/L) and platelet count (8 × 10^9/L). Coagulation parameters were within normal limits. After diagnosis of hemolytic uremic syndrome, treatment included plasma exchange for six days with cryoprecipitate poor plasma. Initially, lab values began to normalize but again began to worsen. Antibiotic treatment was also provided as a result of fever and positive blood cultures for Staphylococcus aureus. After 34 days of hospitalization and two plasmapharesis treatments, the patient was discharged. Prednisone was tapered over a month period and blood counts remained with normal limits during follow-up.

The authors noted that this is the first published case of hemolytic uremic syndrome associated with clopidrogel. Although an exact mechanism of action was not provided, the authors cautioned clinicians to be aware of this potential hematologic toxic effect.

Moy B et al. (Marcoux P, Harvard Vanguard Med Assoc, Dept Hematol-Oncology, 133 Brookline Ave, Boston, MA 02215; e-mail:jmarcoux@bics.bwh.harvard.edu) Hemolytic uremic syndrome associated with clopidogrel. Arch Intern Med 160: 1370–1372 (May 8) 2000

CLOPIDOGREL
Hemolytic Uremic Syndrome

A 70-year-old patient developed thrombocytopenia (43 × 10^9/L) approximately four days after starting clopidogrel (300 mg followed by 75 mg once daily) post transluminal coronary angioplasty. Other chronic medications prior to angioplasty included metoprolol, perindopril, hydrochlorothiazide, nifedipine, simvastatin, and acenocoumarol (no dosages provided). Medications immediately post-angioplasty included abciximab for 12 hours. Acenocoumarol was also continued. Other changes in laboratory values included a decrease in hemoglobin (8.5 vs 4.0 mmol/L) and an increase in lactate dehydrogenase (502 vs 1362 U/L). Significant changes also occurred in values indicative of renal dysfunction, including creatinine level (291 umol/L), urea levels (40.9 mmol/L), urinary sodium excretion (39 mmol/L), and proteinuria (2.8 g/24 hr). However, laboratory screenings and cultures for infectious etiologies were negative. After clopidogrel withdrawal, hemolysis and thrombocytopenia reversed within a few days, and kidney function gradually improved.

The authors concluded that this patient experienced hemolytic uremic syndrome as a result of clopidogrel therapy, based on the temporal relationship between drug administration and appearance of side effects. Although no mechanism of action was provided, the authors suggested that clinicians should be aware of this potential complication.

Oomen PHN et al (Univ Hosp Groningen, NL—9700 RB Groningen, the Netherlands) Hemolytic uremic syndrome in a patient treated with clopidogrel. Ann Intern Med 132:1006 (Jun 20) 2000 (letter)

CLOPIDOGREL
Thrombotic Thrombocytopenic Purpura, Early Article Release

Editor's Note: On April 20, 2000, the *New England Journal of Medicine* released an article (posted on the Internet) prior to the print publication date because of the potential clinical implications. The following article, was published June 15th, and may be found at the url: **http://www.nejm.org/content/bennett/1.asp** Between March 1998 and March 2000, 11 cases of clopidogrel related thrombotic thrombocytopenic purpura was identified (age range: 35 to 79 yrs). Clopidogrel therapy duration ranged from three to 14 days in 10 patients and in three weeks in one patient. Concurrent medications included atorvastatin and simvastatin in five patients. Clinical manifestations were thrombocytopenia and microangiographic hemolytic anemia. In the majority of patients, platelet counts and hematocrit were decreased ($<20,000/mm^3$ and 27%, respectively). Some patients (7) also experienced neurological changes, including disorientation (2), slurred speech (2), confusion (1), aphasia (1), and coma (1). Four patients experienced renal dysfunction. Treatment with plasma exchange (range: 1 to 30) was successful in most patents (10) in reversing symptoms and lab abnormalities. One patient died.

The authors concluded that clopidogrel therapy was associated with related thrombotic thrombocytopenic purpura in these patients. They also cautioned clinicians to be aware of this possible adverse event when prescribing clopidogrel.

Bennett CL et al (VA Chicago Healthcare System, Lakeside Div, Chicago IL 60611; email:cbenne@nwu. edu) Thrombotic thrombocytopenic purpura associated with clopidogrel. N Engl J Med (Jun 15) 2000

DALTEPARIN
Alopecia (First Report*)

A nine-year-old patient developed extensive alopecia 10 weeks after starting subcutaneous dalteparin (100 U/kg twice daily) therapy for right transverse/sigmoid sinus thrombosis. During hospitalization the patient had a right-sided cortical mastoidectomy, removal of the sinus thrombosis, and drainage of the perisinus abscess. Other concurrent medications during hospitalization included third generation cephalosporins, penicillins, aminoglycosides, metoclopramide, acetaminophen, and ibuprofen. Six weeks post surgery the patient's symptoms had improved but dalteparin therapy was continued for an additional month. Within two weeks after dalteparin was discontinued, hair loss improved.

The authors proposed that dalteparin was the cause for alopecia in this patient based on the temporal relationship between drug administration and appearance/disappearance of symptoms. Other drugs that the patient received (e.g., ibuprofen and gentamicin) have also been associated with alopecia. The mechanism of action for anticoagulant induced alopecia is unknown but may be related to premature transformation of growing hairs into a resting phase.

Barnes C et al (Dept Hematology, Royal Children's Hosp, Parkville, Australia) Alopecia and dalteparin: a previously unreported association. Blood 96(4):1618–1619 (Aug 15) 2000 (letter)

EPOETIN ALFA
Cerebral Venous Thrombosis

A 37-year-old patient with end stage renal disease on peritoneal dialysis developed severe headaches after three months of therapy with epoetin alfa. During this time period, the hematocrit increased from 0.27 at the beginning of therapy to 0.55 at the end of the third month, despite decreasing dosages of epoetin from 7000 U to 2500 U at three months. Two weeks after epoetin was stopped the patient developed a severe headache with a hematocrit of 0.49. Upon hospitalization the platelet count was 149×10^9/L. CT cranial scans and MRI tests were consistent with a sinus thrombosis. Intravenous heparin and analgesics were initiated. Recovery was complicated by a retroperitoneal bleed while on heparin therapy. Eventual discharge on warfarin therapy occurred.

The authors noted that this is the first case of cerebral venous thrombosis associated with epoetin alfa therapy possibly related to hyperviscosity due to polycythemia alone or with other risk factors.

Finelli PF & Carley MD (Dept Neurol, Hartford Hosp, 80 Seymour St, Hartford, CT 06102) Cerebral venous thrombosis associated with epoetin alfa therapy. Arch Neurol 57:260–262 (Feb) 2000

EPOETIN ALFA
Pyrogenic Reactions Due to Extrinsic Contamination

On March 24, 2000 the manufacturer of Epogen (Amgen Inc) contacted health professionals regarding postmarketing adverse events, specifically 21 episodes of bacteremia or pyrogenic reactions in patients receiving the product at dialysis units. An investigation by the Centers for Disease Control revealed that unsafe practices resulted in extrinsic bacterial contamination of the used vials. Unused portions of single dose preservative free vials were being collected and pooled into a common vial for use in other patients. This practice was most likely responsible for bacterial contamination and resultant reactions. The manufacturers noted that this product is commercially supplied in single use vials without preservative and any unused portion should be discarded.

21 episodes of bacterial/pyrogenic reactions with Epogen. Amgen Inc (Mar 24) 2000. (http://www.fda.gov/medwatch/safety/2000/epogen.pdf)

HEPARIN
Thrombocytopenia, Legal Action

A patient developed heparin induced thrombocytopenia after receiving heparin pre and perioperatively for cardiac bypass surgery. The diagnosis was not made until eight days post surgery. The plaintiff contended that the late diagnosis of heparin induced thrombocytopenia with thrombosis resulted in amputation of her left arm and several toes. The defendant claimed that platelet counts typically decrease post surgery, that this was not unusual and that heparin therapy was essential prior to and during cardiac surgery. The case was settled prior to trial date by the cardiologist ($170,000), cardiac surgeon ($350,000) and the hospital ($175,000).

E. Falciano & J. Falciano vs Hospital and doctors Heparin induced thrombocytopenia—$695,000 settlement. Med Malpractice, Verdicts, Settlements & Experts 15(11):23 (Nov) 1999

FERROUS SULFATE
Hemosiderosis

After five years of taking excessive iron supplementation (up to 300 mg elemental iron daily) a 10-year-old girl had an elevated serum ferritin (1190 ng/mL) and serum iron with 88% transferrin saturation. Other hematological parameters, such as MCV and hemoglobin values were within normal limits, as were glucose tolerance, thyroid function and cardiac function. A percutaneous liver biopsy revealed mild fibrosis. Analysis of the extracted liver tissue demonstrated an abnormally high iron content (7.9 mg iron/gram dry weight). Elevated liver function tests included aspartate aminotransferase (50 U/L) and alanine aminotransferase (80 U/L). Iron supplementation was discontinued and 10 isovolemic phlebotomies (450 to 500 mL) were performed over a four month period with an estimated iron removal of 4.5 grams. Serum ferritin, serum iron and transferrin saturation decreased post-phlebotomy. Follow-up testing two years later revealed normal oral iron absorption and normal DNA patterns ruling out idiopathic hemochromatosis. Hematological parameters and liver function tests remained within normal ranges over the next 10 years of follow-up.

The authors concluded that this patient developed hemosiderosis as a result of ingesting a large amount of iron over a period of five years. They also suggested that phlebotomy is the most efficient method for removing body iron.

Pearson HA et al (Dept Peds, 333 Cedar St, New Haven CT 06520; e-mail:howardpearson @yale.edu) Hemosiderosis in a normal child secondary to oral iron medication. Pediatrics 105(2):429–431 (Feb) 2000

HEPARIN
Thrombocytopenia, Legal Action

A 63-year-old bypass surgery patient developed thrombocytopenia on the second post-operative day. Platelet counts, rechecked two days later, were extremely low, necessitating heparin withdrawal. Thrombi developed in both legs, ultimately requiring amputation. The plaintiff claimed that heparin should have been stopped after initial decreases in platelets were observed. The defendants maintained that platelet monitoring every other day was standard and outcome would not have differed. A jury awarded $2.29 million dollars.

V Parisi & F Parisi vs B Fein & I Jacobwitz. Failure to monitor platelet count during start of heparin therapy after bypass surgery—thrombocytopenia necessitates amputations on both legs—$2.29 million New York verdict. Med Malprac-tice Verdicts, Settlements & Experts 16(8):20–21 (Aug) 2000

STREPTOKINASE
Adverse Events Related to Unlabeled Usage

On December 10, 1999, the manufacturer of streptokinase (AstraZeneca) contacted health professionals regarding postmarketing adverse events when the agent was used to restore patency of intravenous catheters. The manufacturer noted that this indication was not an FDA approved indication and is not included in the product package information. Serious events reported to the manufacturer and the FDA included hypotension, hypersensitivity reactions, apnea and bleeding. The manufacturer also noted that several of the reports involved the use of high dose streptokinase in small volumes (250,000 IU/2 mL) for catheter occlusion. The manufacturer's letter to health professionals cautioned clinicians to consider the risk of potentially life-threatening reactions associated with the use of streptokinase when used for this purpose. In addition, health care professionals were encouraged to report serious adverse events to the manufacturer and the FDA MedWatch program.

Important safety information—streptokinase health professional letter. AstraZeneca (Dec 10) 1999. (Http://www.fda.gov/medwatch/safety/1999/strept.htm)

TICLOPIDINE
Aplastic Anemia

An 83-year-old woman with coronary artery disease and chronic renal failure was hospitalized for pulmonary edema and chest pain. Upon admission laboratory tests included white blood cell count (1.3×10^9/L), hematocrit (29%) and platelets (153×10^9/L). Medications upon admission included amiloride/HCTZ, diltiazem and ticlopidine (250 mg daily) which was recently added six weeks prior to admission. A bone marrow aspirate revealed aplastic marrow, and despite immediate ticlopidine withdrawal the WBC continued to drop (0.9×10^9/L). Ceftazidime was initiated for left lower pneumonia and 11 days post ticlopidine withdrawal, WBC stabilized (0.9–1.1×10^9/L). G-CSF was started (5 mcg/kg/day) for decreasing platelets (37×10^9/L). Within one week WBC normalized and platelet counts increased. At follow-up post discharge, hematological parameters were within normal ranges.

The authors concluded that ticlopidine was responsible for aplastic anemia in this patient. They also noted that renal failure and advanced age placed her at risk for higher plasma concentrations and possible toxicities. Twenty similar cases from the literature were also reviewed.

Taher A et al. Ticlopidine induced aplastic anemia and quick recovery with G-CSF: Case report and literature review. Am J Hematology 63:90–93 (Feb) 2000

WARFARIN
Submucosal Hemorrhage Mimics Renal Pelvic Tumor
(First Report*)

A 73-year-old woman stabilized on warfarin therapy for four years was hospitalized for gross hematuria and slight lumbago. An IVP revealed irregular right caliceal and pelvic defects and a hydronephrotic left kidney. An abdominal CT scan suggested thickening of the bilateral renal pelvic wall indicative of a renal pelvic or gastric tumor. When repeated, the abdominal CT scan revealed a large hematoma between the gluteus medius and gluteus minimus.

The authors concluded that the bilateral renal pelvic wall thickening allowed hemorrhaging in to the submucosa, imitating a renal pelvic mass. They noted that hemorrhages near the urinary tract typically are retroperitoneal, intraluminal and intrarenal. This is the first report of submucosal hemorrhaging.

Hiratsuka Y et al. Anticoagulant induced submucosal hemorrhage mimicking a renal pelvic tumor. J Urology 163:231 (Jan) 2000

WARFARIN AND CELECOXIB
Interaction: Increased INRs

Increased INRs without clinical bleeding were observed in a 73-year-old inpatient. Medications on admission included chronic therapy (about three years) with captopril (6.25 mg three times daily), furosemide (20 mg daily), digoxin (0.25 mg daily), warfarin (5 mg daily), diltiazem (30 mg three times daily), levothyroxine (0.075 mg daily), trazodone (50 mg daily), and acetaminophen/oxycodone (as needed). Celecoxib was added to the regimen approximately five weeks prior to admission (200 mg daily). Prior to celecoxib, the patient was stabilized on warfarin therapy with INRs in therapeutic range (2.1 to 3.2). However, upon arrival in the emergency room and on the first hospital day, INRs were 4.4 and 5.68, respectively. Both warfarin and celecoxib were discontinued and treatment included fresh frozen plasma (two units) and two subcutaneous vitamin K injections (1 mg each). By hospital day six the patient's INR had decreased to 1.07. Rechallenge with warfarin or celecoxib did not occur.

The authors concluded that celecoxib potentiated the anticoagulant effects of warfarin, possibly via competition of cytochrome P450 metabolism or protein binding displacement. They also suggested that patients on warfarin therapy should be closely monitored when celecoxib is added or withdrawn from the regimen.

Mersfelder TL & Stewart LR (Coll Pharmacy, Ferris State Univ, 220 Ferris Dr, Big Rapids, MI 49307; e-mail:mersfelt@mercyhealth.com) Warfarin and celecoxib interaction. Ann Pharmacother 34:325–327 (Mar) 2000

WARFARIN AND CIPROFLOXACIN
Hypothrombinemia, Bleeding

Two patients experienced clinical bleeding due to hypothrombinemia induced by an interaction between ciprofloxacin and warfarin therapy.

Patient 1: A 50-year-old woman was admitted for lethargy, nausea, frontal headache and dysuria approximately two days after starting oral ciprofloxacin (500 mg twice daily) for a suspected urinary tract infection. Other medications upon admission included prednisone, cyclosporine, lisinopril, methotrexate, diltiazem, folate, conjugated estrogens and warfarin. One week prior to hospitalization she was stabilized on warfarin with INRs and PTs of 3.0 and 20.8, respectively. A CT of the head to investigate confusion revealed bilateral subdural hematomas. At this time, INR and PT were 8.8 and 36.5 seconds. The INR decreased to 1.0 after administration of vitamin K (10 mg). Clot evacuation was successful and the remainder of her hospital stay was uneventful. Six days post discharge, INR was within therapeutic range (2.4) on the previous warfarin dose.

Patient 2: A 56-year-old man, previously stabilized on warfarin therapy was hospitalized for refractory epistaxis approximately four days after starting oral ciprofloxacin (750 mg twice daily) for scrotal cellulitis. Upon admission, his INR and PT were 53.9 and 81.2 seconds, respectively. Other concurrent medications included amiodarone, folate, prednisone, diltiazem, lisinopril, ranitidine, furosemide, digoxin, nabumetone and methotrexate. Bleeding improved over a two day period after treatment with vitamin K (6 mg), fresh frozen plasma (12 units), nasal packing and oxymetazoline nasal spray. However, a surgical wound (post scrotal surgery) continued to bleed, requiring an additional vitamin K injection (4 mg). The INR was 1.0 on post-operative day three. INR was 2.2 on discharge while taking warfarin at previous doses.

A total of 64 similar ciprofloxacin—warfarin cases were obtained from the FDA's Spontaneous Reporting System database in April 1997. These events occurred in patients with median age of 72 yrs and bleeding problems became evident after a median of 5.5 days of ciprofloxacin therapy. The median INR and PT were 10.0 and 38.0 seconds, respectively. Sequaele was serious in 15 cases causing hospitalization, 2 cases noting bleeding and possibly responsible for one death. For the majority of cases, treatment included vitamin K alone, fresh frozen plasma alone or a combination of the two.

The authors concluded that the addition of ciprofloxacin to previously stabilized warfarin therapy was responsible for bleeding in these two patients. Although an exact mechanism of action is not established, possible actions include protein binding, metabolism inhibition or interference with warfarin elimination. Clinicians were encouraged to monitor INR levels within four to five days after starting ciprofloxacin therapy.

Ellis RJ et al (Div Hematology/Oncology, Univ Kansas Med Center, 1417 Bell, 3901 Rainbow Blvd, KC, KS 66160; e-mail:rellis2@kumc.edu) Ciprofloxacin-warfarin coagulopathy: a case series. Am J Hematology 63:28–31 (Jan) 2000

WARFARIN AND FLUOROURACIL
Interaction: Increased Anticoagulation

In a retrospective hospital review over a three year period, five cancer patients who received concurrent warfarin and 5-fluorouracil (5-FU) were identified to examine the possibility of a drug interaction. Prior to chemotherapy, all patients were stabilized on warfarin therapy (INRs: 2-3) and monitored monthly via an anticoagulation clinic. However, after chemotherapy started, patients required a mean reduction of 44% in warfarin dosing to maintain target INRs. In four patients who received full 5-FU doses, warfarin dosage reductions were 50%. The mean warfarin dose prior to and during chemotherapy was 40.66 mg and 24 mg, respectively. Two patients required hospitalization, one for major retroperitoneal bleeding and the other for the administration of fresh frozen plasma.

The authors suggested that this data is indicative of a clinically significant interaction between 5-FU and warfarin and that further prospective controlled trials are needed to determine definitive causality.

Kolesar JM et al (Sch Pharmacy, Univ Wisconsin—Madison, 425 North Charter St, Madison, WI 53706-1515) Warfarin-5FU interaction—a consecutive case series. Pharmacotherapy 19(12):1445–1449 (Dec) 1999

WARFARIN AND GEMCITABINE
Interaction: Increased INRs

A 63-year-old man, previously stabilized on warfarin therapy (57.5 mg weekly), experienced increased INRs (3.52 from 1.94) after receiving the first dose of gemcitabine (2380 mg per week over 30 minutes for three weeks). Other concurrent medications included potassium chloride, digoxin, isosorbide dinitrate, simvastatin, ranitidine, multivitamins, furosemide and diltiazem. During a two-week rest period between gemcitabine cycles, INRs returned to therapeutic range (2.08 to 2.13) once the warfarin dose was reduced (52.5 mg weekly). However, the INR increased again to 3.58 after the second gemcitabine cycle was started, requiring a further reduction in warfarin dosage (50 mg weekly). INRs became subtherapeutic after gemcitabine was discontinued and warfarin doses were gradually increased. Periodic liver function monitoring revealed elevations during chemotherapy cycles.

The authors concluded that decreased warfarin doses were needed because of gemcitabine-induced hepatotoxicity, possibly decreasing warfarin metabolism or synthesis of clotting factors.

Kinikar SA & Kolsear JM (Univ Wisconsin-Madison Sch Pharmacy, 425 North Charter St, Madison, WI 53706–1515) Identification of a gemcitabine-warfarin interaction. Pharmacotherapy 19(11):1331–1333 (Nov) 1999

WARFARIN AND METHYL SALICYLATE (Topical)
Interaction: Anticoagulation Potentiation

A 22-year-old patient previously stabilized on warfarin therapy for one month had elevated INRs (12.2) after applying topical 7% menthol/0.05% methyl salicylate to both knees for eight nights. The patient was not taking any other medications during the previous four weeks. Dietary changes also included increased spinach consumption. Increased bruising and bleeding of the gums after brushing was also observed. Management included oral vitamin K (2.5 mg), holding the next warfarin dose, and stopping gel application. The next INR decreased to 5.0. Reinstitution of warfarin at previous dosages resulted in therapeutic INRs during follow-up monitoring.

The authors concluded that topical salicylate therapy was responsible for anticoagulation potentiation in this patient. Possible mechanisms included systemic salicylate absorption in amounts sufficient to affect vitamin K metabolism or displacement of warfarin via protein binding. Clinicians are encouraged to discuss this interaction with patients who may use topical salicylate products.

Joss JD & LeBlond RF (Dept Pharmaceutical Care, Univ Iowa Health Care, 200 Hawkins Dr, Iowa City, IA 52246; e-mail:jacqueline-joss@uiowa.edu) Potentiation of warfarin anticoagulation associated with topical methyl salicylate. Ann Pharmacother 34:729–733 (Jun) 2000

WARFARIN AND MICONAZOLE (Vaginal) Interaction: Increased Anticoagulation Effect (First Report*)

A 53-year-old woman, previously stabilized on warfarin therapy (45 mg/week) developed bruising on her legs and arms approximately three days after starting vaginal miconazole therapy (200 mg suppositories) for a yeast infection. The only other concurrent medication was mexiletine (200 mg three times daily) for ventricular tachycardia. Prior to miconazole therapy, INRs were stabilized at a mean of 2.69. However, INRs taken on the third and last day of miconazole therapy were significantly elevated (9.77) until warfarin dosing was held for 24 hours (6.93). Rechallenge with miconazole therapy was required due to a persistent vaginal infection. Miconazole vaginal suppositories were restarted at 100 mg daily for seven days. Reduced warfarin dosing (32.5 mg/week) during concurrent therapy resulted in INRs within previous ranges (3.27). After miconazole therapy was discontinued, warfarin dosing was increased to previous dosage levels with subsequent therapeutic INRs.

Approximately one year later, a repeat seven day course of miconazole (100 mg) vaginal therapy was required due to another yeast infection. Despite a 19% reduction in warfarin dosing during concurrent therapy, INRs increased to 7.13. However, evidence of clinical bleeding was absent. INRs returned to 3.72 when warfarin was held for two days.

The authors noted that this is the first published case report of a drug interaction with vaginal miconazole therapy and warfarin. Although only a small amount of vaginal miconazole is thought to reach the systemic circulation, the authors proposed that this drug interfered with previously stable warfarin therapy. Possible proposed mechanisms of action included either a decrease in warfarin clearance or an increase in the plasma free fraction portion of warfarin. The authors encouraged clinicians to be aware of this potentially significant drug interaction and to adjust the warfarin dose accordingly.

Thirton DJG et al (Farquhar Zanetti LA: Anticoagulation Clin Henry Ford Health System, 3500 Fifteen Mile Rd, Sterling Heights, MI 48310) Potentiation of warfarin's hypothrombinemic effect with miconazole vaginal suppositories. Pharmacotherapy 20(1): 98–99 (Jan) 2000

WARFARIN AND NABUMETONE
Anticoagulation Potentiation (First Report*)

A 72-year-old man, previously stabilized on warfarin therapy (34 mg/week) with INRs in therapeutic range (2.0 to 2.1), had an increased INR (3.7) within one week after starting nabumetone therapy (750 mg twice daily). Other chronic medications included digoxin, quinidine, topical nitroglycerin, ranitidine, hyoscyamine, zolpidem and multivitamins. Despite a planned reduction in warfarin dosage the patient developed right knee swelling and pain which was diagnosed as hemarthrosis. Warfarin therapy was discontinued and nabumetone continued. Four days prior to surgical repair of the right knee cartilage, symptoms suggestive of a TIA occurred precipitating the prescribing of clopidrogel while continuing nabumetone. Follow-up at one year revealed that the patient did not have any neurologic events and no further occurrences of hemarthrosis during concurrent therapy.

The authors concluded that increases in INR and hemarthrosis were a result of combined nabumetone and warfarin therapy. Possible mechanisms discussed included warfarin metabolism inhibition and/or protein binding displacement. The authors also recommended that all patients on warfarin therapy should be closely monitored when new therapy is added.

Dennis VC et al. Potentiation of oral anticoagulation and hemarthrosis associated with nabumetone. Pharmacotherapy 20(2):234–239 (Feb) 2000

WARFARIN AND TOLTERODINE
Interaction: Prolonged International Normalized Ratio (INR)

Two cases of prolonged INRs are described in patients on concurrent tolterodine and warfarin therapy.

Patient 1: A 72-year-old man, previously stabilized on warfarin therapy for one year (5 mg daily), developed prolonged INRs (6.1) within two weeks after starting tolterodine therapy (2 mg daily). Other chronic medications included nortriptyline (50 mg nightly), digoxin (0.25 mg daily), sustained release verapamil (120 mg daily) and melatonin (3 mg nightly). INRs had become elevated, requiring dosage omission, during a 56 day course of levofloxacin therapy completed prior to the initiation of tolterodine. Tolterodine was stopped and warfarin doses held for three days, resulting in an INR of 1.2. After reinitiating warfarin dosing at previous levels (5 mg daily) INRs remained in therapeutic ranges.

Patient 2: An 83-year-old man, previously stabilized on warfarin therapy (5 mg daily), developed prolonged INRs (7.4) within 10 days after starting tolterodine therapy for nocturia and bladder discomfort (2 mg daily). Other chronic medications included colchicine (0.6 mg as needed), pikocarpine ocular drops, isosorbide mononitrate (20 mg twice daily), furosemide (20 mg daily), doxazosin (4 mg nightly), and ibuprofen (200 mg weekly). The tolterodine was stopped due to inefficacy and three doses of warfarin were held until INRs normalized. After reinitiating warfarin dosing at previous levels (5 mg daily) INRs remained in therapeutic ranges.

The authors concluded that the temporal course of tolterodine administration and increases in INR suggested a drug interaction with warfarin, resulting in increased anticoagulation. Possible mechanisms of action included cytochrome P450 inhibition and possible protein binding competition. The authors also encouraged increased INR monitoring in patients receiving concurrent therapy with these agents.

Colucci VJ & Rivey MP (Sch Pharmacy, Univ Montana, Missoula, MT 59812; e-mail: colucci@selway.umt.edu) Tolterodine-warfarin drug interaction. Ann Pharmacother 33: 1173–1175 (Nov) 1999

CARDIAC

CARDIAC

CARDIAC

CARDIAC

CARDIAC

CARDIAC

Drug	Interacting Drug	ADR	Page Number
Amiodarone		Lupus	86
Amiodarone		Hyponatremia	85
Amiodarone		Pulmonary toxicity	85
Amiodarone		Blue gray syndrome	87
Captopril		Toxic epidermal necrolysis	87
Cerivastatin		Rhabdomyolysis	88
Cerivastatin	Gemfibrozil	Rhabdomyolysis	89
Digoxin		Glucose intolerance	90
Digoxin		Mesentric infarction^	91
Digoxin	St. John's wort	Digoxin levels decreased	91
Diltiazem		Oral ulcerations*	92
Diltiazem	Simvastatin	Simvastatin concentrations increased	92
Dobutamine		Hand weakness (+)	93
Doxazosin		Priapism*	94
Gemfibrozil	Cerivastatin	Rhabdomyolysis	89
Nifedipine		Hypotension (overdose)	94
Propranolol	Gabapentin	Dystonia	95
Quinapril		Angioneurotic edema	95
Simvastatin	Diltiazem	Simvastatin concentrations increased	92
Verapamil		Oral ulcerations*	92

* = first report
^ = death
(+) = legal action

Cardiac

AMIODARONE
Hyponatremia (Second Report*)

A 62-year-old woman was hospitalized approximately six months after starting amiodarone (300 mg once daily). Symptoms upon admission included tachycardia (100 bpm), irregular heart rate, generalized weakness, nausea, vomiting, and headache. Other chronic concurrent medications included famotidine (40 mg daily) and lorazepam (1 mg daily). Abnormal laboratory values included reduced serum sodium levels (121 mmol/L) and serum osmolality (243 mmol/kg H_2O) with increased urine sodium levels (141 mmol/L). Other laboratory values were within normal ranges including calcium, potassium, serum creatinine, liver enzyme levels, and thyroid function. Prajmalium bitartrate was substituted and serum sodium levels gradually increased and general weakness reversed within five days after amiodarone withdrawal. Within two weeks, serum sodium levels normalized (143 mmol/L) and hyponatremia did not recur.

The authors noted that this is only the second reported case of amiodarone induced hyponatremia in an elderly patient as a result of inappropriate secretion of antidiuretic hormone (SIADH). A mechanism of action was not proposed. The authors encouraged clinicians to be aware of this rare and potential complication associated with amiodarone therapy.

Odeh M et al (PO Box 6477, Hiaja 31063, Israel) Hyponatremia during therapy with amiodarone. Arch Intern Med 159:2599–2600 (Nov 22) 1999

AMIODARONE
Pulmonary Toxicity

Amiodarone induced pulmonary toxicity was reported in two elderly men.

Patient 1: A 77-year-old man developed diaphoresis, hypotension (100/60 mmHg) and tachypnea approximately 15 days after starting amiodarone therapy (maintenance dose: 400 mg daily). Pulmonary examination revealed crackles and decreased airflow. A chest x-ray displayed interstitial and alveolar infiltration with bilateral pleural effusions. Amiodarone therapy was also discontinued at this time. A CT scan of the chest indicated acute amiodarone hypersensitivity pneumonitis. Treatment included intravenous methylprednisolone (80 mg every eight hours), mechanical ventilation and incomplete bronchoscopy with bronchoaveolar lavage. Open lung biopsy revealed diffuse interstitial pneumonitis. His condition gradually deteriorated resulting in eventual death 26 days post hospital admission.

Patient 2: A 72-year-old man was hospitalized with fever, nonproductive cough and dyspnea. His current medications included amiodarone (300 mg daily), ramipril (10 mg daily), and aspirin (325 mg daily). Amiodarone therapy was stopped due to suspected pulmonary toxicity. Chest x-rays revealed interstitial infiltrates without pleural effusions. A CT scan was consistent with amiodarone pneumonitis. Open lung biopsy revealed the presence of infiltrates and fibrous tissue with lymphocytes and plasma cells. Treatment included intubation with short term (three days) intravenous methylprednisolone (500 mg daily) followed by oral prednisone (75 mg daily via nasogastric tube). The patient's condition gradually improved with discharge at three weeks post admission.

The authors concluded that amiodarone was responsible for pulmonary toxicity in both these elderly patients and that the lowest effective dose of amiodarone should be used. They also encouraged clinicians to educate patients about possible early signs and symptoms of pulmonary complications and to report these events as soon as they appear.

Kanji Z et al (Pharmacy Dept, Lions Gate Hosp, 231 E 15th St, North Vancouver, BC, Canada, V7L 2L7) Amiodarone induced pulmonary toxicity. Pharmacotherapy 19(12):1463–1466 (Dec) 1999

AMIODARONE
Lupus

A 71-year-old patient was hospitalized with pleuritic chest pain, dyspnea on exertion and non-productive cough. Medications included amiloride (no dosage provided), digitalis (no dosage provided) and amiodarone (200 mg twice daily) for two years. Upon admission the patient was noted to have a malar rash, aortic systolic murmur and decreased respiratory rate. Abnormal laboratory values included, erythrocyte sedimentation rate (90 mm/h), anemia and positive titers for circulating immune complexes and antinuclear antibodies. Other hematological parameters were within normal limits. Chest x-ray revealed bilateral pleural effusions without fibrotic changes.

Bacterial etiologies were negative. After amiodarone was discontinued the patient's condition gradually improved with a minor relapse at the third week. Recovery was uneventful and ANA titer remained weakly positive.

The authors concluded that amiodarone induced lupus in this patient, causing a relapse due to slow drug elimination from the body. Possible mechanisms included cross-reactivity of the drug and nucleic acids, hapten complex formation between the drug and nucleic acids, or interference with complement pathway via immune cell activation.

Susano R et al (Dept Med, Hosp Central de Asturia, C Julian Claveria s/n, 33006, Oviedo, Spain) Amiodarone induced lupus. Ann Rheum Dis 58:655–666 (Oct) 1999

AMIODARONE
Blue Gray Syndrome

A 69-year-old patient developed a blue gray skin pigmentation on the face, ears, and dorsal side of the forearms during long-term amiodarone therapy for recurrent sustained ventricular tachycardia (400 mg daily). Although previous unsuccessful therapy included quinidine and mexiletine, there were no concurrent medications taken during the development of this skin condition. Pigmentation was not evident on covered areas (e.g., wrist and forehead) and the patient did not describe other symptoms of amiodarone toxicity. The dosage was not changed as this condition was considered benign and other therapeutic alternatives were unlikely.

The authors concluded that this case of photodermatitis was most likely due to amiodarone therapy as a result of deposition of drug in the skin. They also noted that this reaction usually occurs with dosages higher than 200 mg daily and typically reverses with drug withdrawal.

Rogers KC & Wolfe DA (Dept Pharmacy Practice, Sch Pharmacy, Univ Miss Med Center, 2500 N State St, Jackson, MS 32916; e-mail:kcrogers@pharmacy.umsmed.edu) Amiodarone induced blue gray syndrome. Ann Pharmacother 34:1075 (Sep) 2000

CAPTOPRIL
Toxic Epidermal Necrolysis

A 59-year-old woman was rehospitalized within three days after discharge for nausea, vomiting and malaise. During the previous hospitalization for a hypertensive crisis she was initially stabilized on sodium nitroprusside and successfully switched to captopril at a final dose of 200 mg twice daily. Upon readmission, a rash was observed as a diffuse, pruritic erythroderma. Rash symptoms resolved after treatment with intravenous diphenhydramine and fluids and discontinuation of the suspected agent (hydrochlorothiazide). The patient was discharged shortly thereafter. However, one month later, the patient was readmitted with a new rash, described as a diffuse erythroderma, particularly prominent on the face and arms. Abnormal laboratory values indicated severe neutropenia (white blood count: 900/uL) without neutrophils, monocytes or band forms. Treatment included antibiotics for suspected sepsis and oral hydroxyzine (50 mg every six hours) for severe pruritus. Despite withdrawal of captopril at this time, the patient's condition worsened with large blisters developing on the extremities. Subcutaneous G-CSF was initiated at 5 mcg/kg/day (300 mcg) and increased to 350 mcg. Within 48 hours after starting G-CSF therapy, bone marrow recovery began to gradually improve. By the end of the fifth day of therapy, leukocytosis had developed with significant left shift. Amlodipine (10 mg daily) was substituted for captopril prior to discharge. The patient remained asymptomatic during a one-year follow-up period.

The authors proposed that high dose captopril therapy was responsible for agranulocytosis and toxic epidermal necrolysis in this patient. The use of G-CSF to stimulate neutrophil recovery was a factor in early bone marrow recovery.

Winfred RI et al (M. Elnicki, West Virginia Univ Sch Med, Dept Med, PO Box 9160, Morgantown, WV 26505-9214) Captopril induced toxic epidermal necrolysis and agranulocytosis successfully treated with granulocyte colony stimulating factor. Southern Med J 92(9):918–920 (Sep) 1999

CERIVASTATIN
Rhabdomyolysis

A 52-year-old patient was hospitalized for asthenia, muscle weakness and myalgias within three weeks after starting cerivastatin therapy for hypercholesterolemia (0.1 mg daily). Previous therapy had included simvastatin (10 mg daily for two years) without adverse events. Concurrent therapy included prednisone (7.5 mg daily), cyclosporine (200 mg daily), mycophenolate (2 grams daily), and ranitidine (150 mg daily). Abnormal laboratory values included serum creatinine (1 mg/dL), aspartate aminotransferase (709 IU/L), alanine aminotransferase (828 IU/L), gamma-glutamyltransferase (117 IU/L), lactate dehydrogenase (7080 IU/L) and creatine phosphokinase (12,615 IU/L). Therapy included normal saline and sodium bicarbonate to induce diuresis. Abnormal values returned to baseline within 10 days after cerivastatin was discontinued.

The authors noted that although this patient did not exhibit typical muscular symptoms of rhabdomyolysis, laboratory values indicated this diagnosis. They concluded that cerivastatin was most likely responsible for rhabdomyolysis in this patient.

Rodriguez M et al (Hosp Nuestra Senora de Candelaria, 38010 Santa Cruz de Tenerife, Spain) Cerivastatin induced rhabdomyolysis. Ann Intern Med 132(7):598 (Apr 4) 2000 (letter)

CERIVASTATIN AND GEMFIBROZIL
Rhabdomyolysis

A 64-year-old patient was hospitalized with severe muscle pain and an elevated serum creatine kinase concentration (>16,000 units/L). Three weeks prior to admission cerivastatin (0.3 mg daily) was substituted for colestipol (5 grams/day). Other concurrent therapy included gemfibrozil (300 mg twice daily), atenolol (50 mg twice daily), verapamil (180 mg extended release daily), ibuprofen (400 mg three times daily), lisinopril-HCTZ (10 mg/12.5 mg daily), estriopipate (0.625 mg daily) and aspirin or acetaminophen as needed. Two weeks after starting cerivastatin, the patient developed severe general myalgias, particularly in the right shoulder and arm. Symptoms persisted despite discontinuation of the cerivastatin and gemfibrozil three days prior to hospitalization. Physical examination and most laboratory values upon admission were unremarkable except for an elevated aspartate transaminase (608 u/L) and alanine transaminase (396 u/L). Other elevated tests included serum creatine kinase (>16,000 units/L) with an elevated CK-MB fraction (248.2 ng/mL) and myoglobin concentration (>1000 ng/mL). Rhabdomyolysis was diagnosed. Treatment with rehydration and urinary alkalinzation was beneficial. Creatine kinase decreased to 1573 u/L the day after discharge with a further reduction to 70 u/L at 11 days post-discharge. New antilipemic therapy included colestipol (2 grams three times daily) and atorvastatin (10 mg daily) without further event.

The authors concluded that the development of rhabdomyolysis in this patient was most likely caused by combination therapy with cerivastatin and gemfibrozil. The combination of gemfibrozil with other statin agents has also been responsible for rhabdomyolysis.

Bermingham RP et al (Scalley RD, 3017 Parkview Ct, Ft Collins, CO 80525; e-mail: rds@libra.pvh.org) Rhabdomyolysis in a patient receiving the combination of cerivastatin and gemfibrozil. Am J Health Syst Pharm 57:461–464 (Mar 1) 2000

CERIVASTATIN AND GEMFIBROZIL
Rhabdomyolysis, Renal Failure

A 63-year-old patient developed anuria, severe muscle weakness and was unable to walk. Symptoms began approximately one week after cerivastatin (0.3 mg daily) was added to his regimen. Concurrent medications included gemfibrozil (600 mg daily), aspirin (325 mg daily), ramipril (2.5 mg daily), glicazide (80 mg twice daily), and isosorbide mononitrate (60 mg daily). Renal function, which was previously normal, deteriorated and required hemodialysis. The creatinine level upon admission was 6.6 mg/dL. Other abnormal values included urea (360 mg/dL), uric acid (13.6 mg/dL), and creatine phosphokinase (30,000 mg/dL). An electrocardiogram revealed an acute myocardial infarction. Despite hemodialysis, the patient's condition worsened with subsequent cardiopulmonary arrest and eventual death.

The authors noted that this is only the second report of severe rhabdomyolysis associated with cerivastatin and gemfibrozil combination therapy.

Ozdemir O et al (SSK Bloklari 62/6, Demetevler 06200, Ankara, Turkey; e-mail: drozdemir@yahoo.com) A case of severe rhabdomyolysis and renal failure associated with cerivastatin—gemfibrozil combination therapy. Angiology 51(8):695–697 (Aug) 2000

DIGOXIN
Glucose Intolerance

Three patients with type 2 diabetes mellitus developed better glucose control after digoxin therapy was discontinued. All patients had significant decreases in blood glucose levels, requiring reductions in drugs to treat diabetic conditions.

Patient 1: A 66-year-old woman with a 10 year history of diabetes mellitus developed significantly reduced blood glucose levels during the first few weeks after chronic digoxin therapy was stopped. Dosages for chronic diabetes medications had gradually increased over the last year and included insulin (164 IU daily), metformin (1500 mg daily) and glibenclamide (3.5 mg daily). Other medications included digoxin (0.25 mg daily). After digoxin was stopped, glucose changes were significant enough to require a dosage reduction for insulin (114 IU daily) and metformin (500 mg daily). Metformin was eventually discontinued. Glibenclamide dosages remained unchanged. At a 14-month follow-up, fasting blood glucose levels were stabilized on insulin (104 IU daily) and glibenclamide (3.5 mg daily).

Patient 2: A 78-year-old diabetic required drastic dosage reductions in insulin requirements after long term digoxin therapy was stopped. Initial regimens while on digoxin therapy (0.25 mg daily) included insulin (72 IU daily) and metformin (2550 mg daily). Post digoxin withdrawal, insulin requirements were decreased to 46 IU daily. Metformin dosage was unchanged. A one-year follow-up period revealed that blood glucose values were stabilized on this regimen.

Patient 3: An 81-year-old diabetic experienced significant improvements in glucose control after digoxin therapy (0.13 mg daily) was stopped for spontaneous conversion of atrial fibrillation into sinus rhythm. Other medications at the time included glibenclamide (14 mg daily). Post digoxin withdrawal fasting morning glucose values decreased from 8–10 mmol/L to 3.0 mmol/L. When digoxin was restarted six weeks later, glucose levels increased to 9–10 mmol/L. At two months fasting morning blood glucose decreased to 4.5 mmol/L most likely caused by a 3.5 kg weight loss. The patient later died of cardiovascular complications.

The authors concluded that in all three patients, changes in blood glucose values were related to changes in digoxin regimens. They noted that the onset of glucose intolerance was gradual while on digoxin therapy and was possibly misinterpreted as disease progression. They suggested that digoxin (and other cardiac glycosides) possibly impairs glucose transport as a result of increased cardiac muscle tone. They encouraged prescribers to be aware that digoxin may have unpredictable results on blood glucose concentrations.

Spigset O & Mjorndal T (Dept Clin Pharmacol, Regional & Univ Hosp, Trondheim, Norway) Increased glucose intolerance related to digoxin treatment in patients with type 2 diabetes mellitus. J Internal Med 246:419–422 (Oct) 1999 (letter)

DIGOXIN
Fatal Non-occlusive Mesenteric Infarction

A 79-year-old patient was hospitalized for digoxin toxicity (4.9 ng/mL). Other medications included amiodarone (200 mg daily) and aspirin (100 mg daily). Despite holding the antiarrhythmic drugs and intravenous saline infusion, the digoxin level remained elevated four days later (2.17 ng/mL). Potassium levels were elevated (5.4 mmol/L) but echocardiography demonstrated good left ventricular systolic function, and abdominal x-ray was normal. Mechanical ventilation was performed. The patient died within a few hours after hospitalization. Autopsy revealed massive infarction of the small bowel.

The authors noted that mesenteric infarction is a rare complication of digoxin intoxication, due to potent vasoconstrictor effects of glycosides on the splanchnic arteries and arterioles.

Guglielminotti J et al (Hopital St Antoine, Assist Pub Hop de Paris, 184 rue du Faubourg St. Antoine, 75571 Paris Cedex 12, France) Fatal non-occlusive infarction following digoxin intoxication. Intensive Care Med 26(6):829 (Jun) 2000 (letter)

DIGOXIN AND ST JOHN'S WORT
Interaction: Decreased Digoxin Levels

In a single blinded, placebo controlled parallel study, 25 healthy volunteers (mean age: 26 yrs) received an oral loading dose of digoxin (0.25 mg twice daily) for two days followed by once daily dosing for an additional 13 days. Steady state serum concentrations were collected on day five and patients were then allocated to receive either placebo or St. John's Wort three times daily for 10 days. Each enteric-coated active treatment tablet contained hypericin (92 mcg), pseudo hypericin (262 mcg) and hyperforin (18.37 mcg). After combination therapy for 10 days, mean half-life (42.8 vs 39.5 hrs) and median time to maximum concentrations (1 hr) were not different when compared to digoxin therapy alone. However, AUC values were decreased by 25 (17.2 vs 12.9 mcg/h/L), Cmax was decreased by 26 (1.9 vs 1.4 mcg/L) and trough concentrations were decreased by 19 (0.58 vs 0.47 mcg/L). In contrast, the AUC values of hypericin and pseudo hypericin were unchanged when administered alone or with digoxin.

The authors concluded that St. John's Wort might reduce the efficacy of digoxin via lowered AUC levels and trough concentrations. They theorized that digoxin kinetics are altered by hypericin extract induced P-glycoprotein activity.

Johne A et al (I Roots, Instit of Clin Pharmacol, Charite, Humboldt Univ of Berlin, Schumannstrasse 20/21, D-10098 Berlin, Germany) Pharmacokinetic interaction of digoxin with an herbal extract from St. John's Wort (hypericum perforatum). Clin Pharmacol & Ther 66:338–345 (Oct) 1999

DILTIAZEM AND SIMVASTATIN
Interaction: Increased Serum Simvastatin Concentrations

In a fixed order study, 10 healthy volunteers received simvastatin alone (single dose: 20 mg) and after two weeks of therapy with sustained release diltiazem (120 mg twice daily). A two week washout period separated the phases. Diltiazem significantly increased several mean simvastatin kinetic parameters, including half-life (1.7 vs 3.9 hrs), maximum concentration (15.9 vs 4.4 ng/mL), and AUC (55.4 vs 11.5 ng/mL/hr). However, median time to peak concentration was not affected (1.5 hrs). Peak concentrations of simvastatin acid was also increased when diltiazem was given concurrently (4.2 vs 1.4 ng/mL). Median time to peak concentration was not affected (3 hrs).

The authors concluded that diltiazem significantly increased the serum concentrations of simvastatin via CYP3A isoenzyme inhibition. They also suggested that this combination should be used with caution in the clinical setting.

Mousa O et al (Hall SD, Wishard Mem Hosp, West Outpatient Bldg, 320, 1001 West Tenth St, Indianapolis, IN 46202–2879; e-mail:sdhall@iupui.edu) The interaction of diltiazem with simvastatin. Clin Pharmacol Ther 67:267–274 (Mar) 2000

DILTIAZEM, VERAPAMIL
Oral Ulcerations (First Report*)

Two patients developed painful oral ulcerations refractory to treatment during oral calcium channel blocker therapy.

Patient 1: An 81-year-old man developed a solitary painful tongue ulceration (1 × 2 cm) which developed at the same time amoxicillin/clavulanate therapy (500 mg three times daily) was initiated for a sinus and ear infection. Other medications included diltiazem (240 mg dally), which was started two months prior to the onset of the ulcer. Medications started after the ulcer developed included HCTZ/losartan (50 mg daily), terazosin and lorazepam. At the time of medical examination the ulcer had persisted for approximately three months. Treatment with oral prednisone and topical fluocinonide gel (0.05%) was unsuccessful. Biopsy of the ulcer revealed nonspecific etiology with intense monocyte infiltration consisting of lymphocytes and plasma cells. Two weeks after diltiazem was stopped the ulcer had almost completely healed and pain was reduced.

Patient 2: A 71-year-old woman sought medical attention for painful tongue ulcerations during the previous three to four years. Chronic medications included captopril (100 mg twice daily) and verapamil (180 to 240 mg daily) for five years. Other medications included oxazepam, metoclopramide, estrogen replacement therapy, thyroxine, and aspirin/caffeine tablets. Biopsies revealed nonspecific ulcerations with mixed inflammatory cell infiltration. Prior laser ablation was only temporarily successful with ulceration recurrence within two weeks. The ulcerations were also refractory to treatment with topical steroids (fluocinonide acetonide and clobetasol propionate) and only mildly abated after the discontinuation of captopril. However, the lesion completely healed within two weeks after verapamil was stopped. A few months later, oral ulceration recurred within 10 days after diltiazem was started. Once again, the lesions reversed after calcium channel blocker therapy was stopped.

The authors concluded that calcium channel blockers were responsible for the first reports of oral ulcerations in these patients. They also noted that captopril may have contributed but was not solely responsible for the ulceration in the second patient. They encouraged clinicians to consider drug-induced etiology in patients who have ulcerations, which are refractory to conventional treatments.

Cohen DM et al (Dept Oral Biology, Univ Nebraska Med Center, Coll of Dentistry, Lincoln, NE) Recalcitrant oral ulcers caused by calcium channel blockers: diagnosis and treatment considerations. JADA 130:1611–1618 (Nov) 1999

DOBUTAMINE
Infiltration, Hand Weakness and Swelling, Legal Action

A 50-year-old hospital patient experienced an infiltrated dobutamine infusion during an intensive care unit admission for cardiopulmonary arrest. Initially, weakness developed in the first, second and third digits of the dominant hand, and despite good recovery, minimal decreased sensation persisted. The plaintiff alleged that inadequate monitoring of the dobutamine infusion resulted in delayed recognition of the problem. The defendants claimed that decreased hand sensation was not related to the dobutamine infiltration but most likely a result of carpal tunnel syndrome. A $50,000 settlement was reached.

Ramsey ML vs Richmond Heights Gen Hosp. Woman blames IV infiltration for swelling and weakness in hand—hospital blames carpal tunnel syndrome—$50,000 Ohio settlement. Med Malpractice, Verdicts, Settlements & Experts 16(5):23 (May) 2000

DOXAZOSIN
Priapism (First Report*)

A 66-year-old man was hospitalized for priapism after increasing his dose of doxazosin from 4 mg daily to 8 mg daily. No other concurrent medications were taken at the time of this event. A transglandular cavernosum-spongiosum shunt was surgically created. Within one month after doxazosin was discontinued he reported return of normal sexual function.

The authors concluded that doxazosin was responsible for this patient's priapism because of an absence of other causes and the temporal sequence of the drug and event. They cautioned clinicians to be aware of this possible reaction as this class of drugs is frequently used to treat benign prostatic hypertrophy.

Avisrror MU et al (Centro Reg de Farmacovigilancia de Castilla y Leon, Instit de Farmacoepidemiologica, Facultad de Med, Valladolid, Spain) Doxazosin and priapism. J Urology 163:238 (Jan) 2000 (letter)

NIFEDIPINE (Overdose)
Prolonged Hypotension

A 14-year-old girl was admitted to the emergency room after ingesting 350 mg of slow release nifedipine (6.4 mg/kg). Upon admission, she was hypotensive (90/44 mmHg), tachypneic (60/min), tachycardic (138 beats/min), and dizzy with a regular heart beat. Immediate treatment in the emergency room included intravenous normal saline infusion and activated oral charcoal infusion (500 mL). Persistent hypotension required additional boluses of normal saline with plasma expanders and calcium chloride injection (18.3 mg/kg) in an intensive care setting. Blood pressures remained low despite further treatment with intravenous dopamine (10 to 20 mcg/kg/min). However, the addition of intravenous norepinephrine (0.3 mcg/kg/min) resulted in gradual blood pressure stabilization allowing tapering of both dopamine and norepinephrine over the next 18 to 28 hours. Once hemodynamically stabilized, the patient's recovery was uneventful with eventual discharge three days after admission.

The authors noted that the hypotensive effect of a nifedipine overdose was prolonged in this patient. They also observed that there is limited published data available regarding the toxicity and management of calcium channel blocker overdose in children.

Cavagnaro F et al (Dept Pediatrics & Poison Center, Catholic Univ Sch Med, Santiago, Chile) A suicide attempt with an oral calcium channel blocker. Vet Human Toxicol 42(2):99–100 (Apr) 2000

PROPRANOLOL AND GABAPENTIN
Dystonia

A 68-year-old patient developed paroxysmal dystonia in both hands approximately two days after propranolol (80 mg daily) was added to gabapentin therapy (900 mg daily) for essential tremor. Although previous unsuccessful therapy included primidone and clonazepam, no other concurrent medications were provided. Dystonic episodes lasted approximately one minute. Other neurological testing, laboratory values, electrolytes and hormonal levels, however, were within normal ranges. The abnormal movements rapidly resolved after the propranolol dosage was reduced (40 mg daily). Combined gabapentin and propranolol therapy was uneventful.

The authors suggested that a synergistic effect occurred between propranolol and gabapentin therapy causing abnormal movements. They proposed that propranolol may have stimulated gabapentin modulation pathways.

Palomeras E et al (Unit Neurologia, Hosp de Mataro, Carratera Cirera, s/n 08304, Mataro, Spain; email: neurologia2@csm.scs.es) Dystonia in a patient treated with propranolol and gabapentin. Arch Neurol 57:570–571 (Apr) 2000

QUINAPRIL
Angioneurotic Edema and Airway Obstruction

A 48-year-old obese man developed significant edema of the neck and face accompanied by drooling within five hours after a transurethral resection of bladder cancer. Intraoperative medications included midazolam (total dose: 3 mg), intravenous fentanyl (100 mcg) and propofol (25 to 75 mcg/kg/min). Maintenance medications administered up to the day of surgery included quinapril (10 mg daily), hydrochlorothiazide (25 mg daily), sertraline (100 mg daily) and alprazolam (0.25 mg daily). These medications were not given during the immediate post-operative recovery period. Progressive symptoms worsened to stridor and other signs of upper airway obstruction, requiring treatment with subcutaneous epinephrine (0.5 mg) and intravenous diphenhydramine (50 mg). Tracheotomy was performed to gain respiratory access and mechanical ventilation. Additional therapy included diphenhydramine (50 mg) and intravenous hydrocortisone (100 mg).

Edema resolved approximately 48 hrs after quinapril was discontinued. Further recovery was uneventful.

The authors attributed this patient's upper airway obstruction a result of a late-onset attack of quinapril induced angioneurotic edema. The patient had been taking the drug for approximately 13 months without event and may have been precipitated by respiratory instrumentation during surgery. They cautioned all clinicians to be aware of this possible adverse event.

Mchaourab A et al (Dept Anesthesiol, Med Coll Wisconsin, 8701 Watertown Plank Rd, Milwaukee WI, 53226; e-mail:alimch@mcw.edu) Airway obstruction due to late onset angioneurotic edema from angiotensin converting enzyme inhibition. Can J Anesthesia 46:975–978 (Oct) 1999

CNS

CNS

CNS

CNS

CNS

CNS

Drug	Interacting Drug	ADR	Page Number
Analgesic-NSAIDS			
Acetaminophen		Anaphylactoid reaction	101
Celecoxib	Warfarin	Coagulation changes	103
Celecoxib		Pancreatitis	103
Celecoxib		Auditory hallucinations	102
Celecoxib		Gastropathy, hypothrombinemia	101
Diclofenac		Aspetic meningitis (recurrent)	104
Diclofenac		Infertility (reversible)	104
Ibuprofen		Renal failure^ (+)	105
Indomethacin		Femoral avascular necrosis	106
Ketoprofen (topical)		Acute renal failure*	106
Meloxicam		Erythema multiforme	107
Nabumetone	Warfarin	INR increased*	107
NSAIDs		CHF in elderly	108
Rofecoxib		Renal failure in transplant patient*	108
Analgesic-Opiates			
Fentanyl	Ritonavir	Fentanyl clearance decreased	109
Fentanyl		Overdose due to heated patch^ (+)	109
Meperidine	Ritonavir	Meperidine concentrations increased	110
Meperidine		Hypertensive crisis	110
Methadone	Ritonavir	Methadone effect decreased	111
Morphine		Self dosing pump error, resp arrest(+)	111
Anticonvulsants			
Carbamazepine		Systemic lupus erythematosus	112
Carbamazepine		Multiple sclerosis exacerbation	112
Divalproex Sodium		Thermoregulatory dysfunction*	113
Gabapentin		Asterixis	114
Gabapentin	Propranolol	Dystonia	115

Drug	Interacting Drug	ADR	Page Number
Lamotrigine		Disseminated intravascular coagulation	115
Lamotrigine		Rash (photosensitivity)	116
Lamotrigine		Agranulocytosis*	116
Phenytoin		Fatal hypersensitivity syndrome^	117
Phenytoin		Intravenous site reactions	117
Valproate		Intravenous site reactions	117
Valproate		Polycystic ovaries, hypogonadism	118
Valproic acid		Pulmonary hemorrhage^	119
Valproic acid		Pancreatitis	120
Vigabatrin		Visual loss	121
Antidepressants			
Amitriptyline		Arrythmias, seizures	122
Amitriptyline	Venlafaxine	Serotonin syndrome	130
Amitriptyline		Cardiac abnormalities	122
Amitriptyline		Hypersensitivity reaction*	123
Bupropion		Overdose: cardiotoxicity	123
Buspirone	Fluoxetine	Serotonin syndrome*	124
Fluoxetine		Pheochromocytoma precipitation*	124
Fluoxetine	Buspirone	Serotonin syndrome*	124
Milnacipran		Raynaud's syndrome	125
Nefazodone	Trazodone	Serotonin syndrome*	125
Paroxetine		Hyponatremia	126
Paroxetine	Risperidone	Serotonin syndrome*	127
Paroxetine		Mydriasis	126
Reboxetine		Hyponatremia	128
Sertraline		Mydriasis	126
SSRIs		Upper GI bleeding: increased risk	128
Trazodone	Nefazodone	Serotonin syndrome*	125
Venlafaxine		Bruxism*	129
Venlafaxine	Amitriptyline	Serotonin syndrome	130
Venlafaxine	Trifluoperazine	Neuroleptic malignant syndrome*	129
Antipsychotics			
Antipsychotics		Heart block (fetal/neonatal)	131
Chlorpromazine		Corneal deposits, cataracts	131
Clozapine		Intersitital nephritis*	132
Clozapine		Stuttering	132
Clozapine		Weight gain, hyperlipidemia	135
Clozapine		Priapism (recurrent)	134
Clozapine		Venous thromboembolism	133
Clozapine		Diabetes mellitus	133
Haloperidol		Medication error, overdose (+)	135

Drug	Interacting Drug	ADR	Page Number
Haloperidol	Imipenem	Hypotension	136
Lithium		Asthma precipitation upon drug withdrawal*	136
Olanzapine		Weight gain	137
Olanzapine		Priapism (recurrent)	134
Risperidone		Hepatotoxicity	138
Risperidone		Blepharospasms	137
Risperidone		Tardive dyskinesia	138
Risperidone	Paroxetine	Serotonin syndrome	127
Thioridazine		QT Prolongation	139
Trifluoperazine	Venlafaxine	Neuroleptic malignant syndrome*	129
Sedative/Hypnotics			
Diazepam		Propylene glycol toxicity	139
Midazolam		Delayed side effects (children)	141
Midazolam		Paradoxical reactions	140
Zolpidem		CNS effects	142
Miscellaneous			
Cyclobenzaprine		Hallucinations	143
Naltrexone		Opioid withdrawal syndrome	143

* = first report
^ = death
(+) = legal action

CNS

ANALGESICS-NSAIDS
ACETAMINOPHEN
Anaphylactoid Reaction

A 65-year-old inpatient became anxious, flushed, weak and short of breath within 30 minutes after receiving acetaminophen (1 gram). Other medications during hospitalization included flucloxacillin, calcitriol, calcium carbonate, and glicazide (no dosages provided). The patient had a previous history of a similar reaction four years prior to this event. Other symptoms during this episode also included dyspnea, hypotension (85/50 mmHg), tachycardia (130 bpm), and inspiratory crackles. Treatment included oxygen and intravenous colloid.

The authors concluded that this patient experienced anaphylaxis related to acetaminophen administration. The authors also noted that although acetaminophen related hepatotoxicity is well known, the incidence of acetaminophen induced anaphylaxis is rare.

Ayonrinde OT & Saker BM. (Royal Perth Hosp, GPO Box X2213, Perth, Western Australia 6000, Australia; e-mail:oyekayon@rph.health.wa.gov.au) Anaphylactoid reactions to paracetamol. Postgrad Med J 76:501–502 (Aug) 2000

CELECOXIB
Hypoprothrombinemia, Gastropathy

A 71-year-old patient was hospitalized with black, tarry, loose stools approximately seven days after starting celecoxib (100 mg twice daily) for arthritis of the hips. Other chronic concurrent medications included warfarin, cimetidine, isosorbide mononitrate, fosinopril, furosemide, digoxin, gemfibrozil, carvedilol, colchicine, and trazodone for about six months. Other symptoms also included weakness, nausea, and melena. INRs for the preceding 12 months prior to celecoxib therapy were within therapeutic range (1.9 to 2.9). However, one week after celecoxib was initiated, the INR was 4. Warfarin and celecoxib were discontinued. Treatment included three units of fresh frozen plasma and initiation of omeprazole. An endoscopic examination revealed a stomach ulcer and diffuse hemorrhagic gastropathy. Recovery was uneventful and the patient was discharged six days later. Warfarin was restarted without further event.

The authors noted that this patient was on several drugs, which are metabolized by the cytochrome P-450 system. They suggested that the addition of celecoxib to warfarin therapy interfered with the cytochrome P-450 system, resulting in increased levels of warfarin, inducing hypoprothombinemia. In addition, they suggested that the role of celecoxib as cause of hemorrhagic gastropathy should be further studied.

Linder JD et al (Wilcox CM, Div of Gastroenterol & Hepatol, 633 ZRB, UAB Station, Birmingham, AL 35294) Cyclooxygenase—2 inhibitor celecoxib: a possible cause of gastropathy and hypoprothrombinemia. S Med J 93(9):930–932 (Sep) 2000

CELECOXIB
Auditory Hallucinations

A 78-year-old patient developed auditory hallucinations within 10 days after starting celecoxib therapy for osteoarthritis (200 mg twice daily). Initial symptoms included thumping sounds, which progressed to voices and hearing repetitive words from the radio and television. Other chronic medications included quinapril (240 mg daily), sustained release verapamil (20 mg twice daily), isosorbide dinitrate (20 mg daily), tamoxifen (20 mg daily) and calcium carbonate (500 mg three times daily). Although a general medicine and otolaryngological examination were unremarkable, celecoxib was discontinued after a psychiatric evaluation. Symptoms improved with total resolution at four days after celecoxib withdrawal. Because of persistent pain, however, the drug was restarted at a lower dose (100 mg twice daily). Symptoms recurred within five days. Discontinuing the drug resulted in symptom improvement. The patient continued to take celecoxib on an intermittent basis with occasional but tolerable auditory hallucinations.

The authors concluded that celecoxib, a cyclooxygenase-2 inhibitor, was responsible for auditory hallucinations in this patient, based on the temporal relationship between administration and appearance and resolution of symptoms. Although a mechanism of action was not provided the authors noted that cyclooxygenase-2 is present in brain tissue.

Lantz MS & Giambanco V (New York, New York) Acute onset of auditory hallucinations after initiation of celecoxib therapy. Am J Psychiatry 157(6):1022–1023 (Jun) 2000 (letter)

CELECOXIB
Acute Pancreatitis

An 81-year-old man was hospitalized with right upper quadrant pain, which developed two days after starting celecoxib (200 mg daily). Chronic concurrent therapy included carbamazepine, trimethoprim-sulfamethoxazole, 1.25 dihydroxycholecalciferol, and levothyroxine (no dosages provided). Upon admission, abnormal laboratory values included serum amylase (6960 U/L), serum lipase (15,100 U/L), calcium (7.7 mg/dL), and serum creatinine (4.7 mg/dL). Amylase and lipase levels were significantly reduced but still in abnormal range five days after admission and calcium levels had normalized. Abdominal tomography revealed an enlarged pancreas accompanied by edema and inflammation. Despite symptom reversal within three days, the patient later died of gastrointestinal hemorrhage and renal failure.

The authors suggested that the coadministration of trimethoprim-sulfamethoxazole and/or carbamazepine may have contributed to the pancreatitis associated with celecoxib in this patient.

Baciewicz Am et al (Univ Hosp Cleveland, Cleveland, OH 44106) Acute pancreatitis associated with celecoxib. Ann Intern Med 132(8):680 (Apr 18) 2000 (letter)

CELECOXIB AND WARFARIN
Interaction: Increased INRs

Increased INRs without clinical bleeding were observed in a 73-year-old inpatient. Medications on admission included chronic therapy (about three years) with captopril (6.25 mg three times daily), furosemide (20 mg daily), digoxin (0.25 mg daily), warfarin (5 mg daily), diltiazem (30 mg three times daily), levothyroxine (0.075 mg daily), trazodone (50 mg daily), and acetaminophen/oxycodone (as needed). Celecoxib was added to the regimen approximately five weeks prior to admission (200 mg daily). Prior to celecoxib, the patient was stabilized on warfarin therapy with INRs in therapeutic range (2.1 to 3.2). However, upon arrival in the emergency room and on the first hospital day, INRs were 4.4 and 5.68, respectively. Both warfarin and celecoxib were discontinued and treatment included fresh frozen plasma (two units) and two subcutaneous vitamin K injections (1 mg each). By hospital day six the patient's INR had decreased to 1.07. Rechallenge with warfarin or celecoxib did not occur.

The authors concluded that celecoxib potentiated the anticoagulant effects of warfarin, possibly via competition of cytochrome P450 metabolism or protein binding displacement. They also suggested that patients on warfarin therapy should be closely monitored when celecoxib is added or withdrawn from the regimen.

Mersfelder TL & Stewart LR (Coll Pharmacy, Ferris State Univ, 220 Ferris Dr, Big Rapids, MI 49307; e-mail:mersfelt@mercyhealth.com) Warfarin and celecoxib interaction. Ann Pharmacother 34:325–327 (Mar) 2000

DICLOFENAC
Recurrent Aseptic Meningitis

Two days after starting an extended release diclofenac product for back pain, a 30-year-old man was hospitalized for headache, nausea, neck pain and photophobia. Laboratory values upon admission revealed an opaque cerebrospinal fluid with an opening pressure greater than 300 mm, protein concentration of 1.2 g/L and CSF:blood glucose ratio of 0.51. Tests for infectious etiologies were negative. However, the patient had a history of aseptic meningitis related to nonsteroidal anti-inflammatory (NSAID) use (naproxen, piroxicam and diclofenac) with four episodes documented within the previous six years. In the last three admissions, symptom onset occurred as short as three days after starting diclofenac. The patient was advised to avoid all NSAIDs and aseptic meningitis did not recur during a two-year follow-up period.

The authors proposed that a possible hypersensitivity reaction involving the meninges might have contributed to this patient's repeated development of aseptic meningitis.

Seaton RA & France AJ (Infection & Immunodeficiency Unit, Kings Cross Hosp, Tayside Univ Hosp, NHS Trust, Dundee DD3 SEA, UK) Recurrent aseptic meningitis following a nonsteroidal anti-inflammatory drug—a reminder. Postgrad Med J 75: 771–772 (Dec) 1999

DICLOFENAC
Reversible Infertility

Four cases are reported of women with severe arthritis undergoing extensive evaluation and treatment of infertility during chronic nonsteroidal anti-inflammatory drug (NSAID) therapy.

Patient 1: A 27-year-old woman was unsuccessfully evaluated and treated for infertility for several years. In addition, intrauterine insemination treatment was unsuccessful. Medications included long term diclofenac (no dosage provided) for six years for severe rheumatoid arthritis-lupus. After diclofenac was discontinued, one cycle of in vitro fertilization was successful, resulting in pregnancy and full term birth. However, further attempts at natural pregnancy were unsuccessful during a four-year period after diclofenac was restarted. Once again, after diclofenac was discontinued, one cycle of in vitro fertilization was successful, resulting in pregnancy and full term birth.

Patient 2: A 41-year-old woman with secondary infertility had three previous normal pregnancies but was unable to conceive during a three year period while taking hydroxychloroquine and diclofenac (no dosages provided) for rheumatoid arthritis. Within five months after discontinuing diclofenac, conception was successful followed by a full term delivery.

Patient 3: A 32-year-old woman was evaluated for infertility five years after starting diclofenac therapy (no dosages provided) for rheumatoid arthritis. Diclofenac was discontinued and ovulation induction was started with clomiphene citrate. Pregnancy occurred after stopping the NSAID and completing three cycles of clomiphene therapy. Although pregnancy was uneventful the fetus died unexpectedly at 36 weeks. Although a subsequent pregnancy also resulted in fetal death at 15 weeks, a third pregnancy was successful.

Patient 4: A 30-year-old woman was evaluated for unexplained infertility during chronic diclofenac therapy (no dosages provided) for rheumatoid arthritis-lupus. Within six months after stopping diclofenac therapy, conception was successful, resulting in a normal delivery at 40 weeks gestation.

The authors suggested that NSAIDs may be responsible for some cases of infertility, possibly interfering with the release of the mature ovum as a result of interfering with prostaglandin synthesis. They also recommended that patients with rheumatological conditions and unexplained infertility should be interviewed for potential NSAID usage.

Mendonca LLF et al (Khamashata MA, Lupus Research Unit, The Rayne Instit, St. Thomas Hosp, London SE1 7EH, UK) Nonsteroidal anti-inflammatory drugs as a possible cause for reversible infertility. Rheumatology 39:880–882 (Sep) 2000

IBUPROFEN
Long Term Therapy without Renal or Hepatic Monitoring, Fatal End Stage Renal Failure, Legal Action

A patient received 2.4 grams of ibuprofen daily for ten years to treat tendonitis in the knee. Throughout this ten year period, liver or renal function monitoring was not performed. Approximately 12 years after starting this regimen, the patient developed acute interstitial nephritis, requiring steroid therapy. Eventually the problem progressed to end stage renal failure, requiring dialysis three times weekly. The patient was unable to receive a kidney transplant prior to her death. The plaintiff claimed that long term ibuprofen therapy without monitoring was negligent. The defendant claimed that long term ibuprofen therapy was not responsible for this patient's end stage renal failure and death. The reported settlement of $375,000 was reached.

Doe J vs Roe R. 2400 milligrams of ibuprofen a day for ten years prescribed without testing of liver and kidney function—end stage renal disease leads to death—$375,000 Connecticut settlement. Med Malpractice Verdicts, Settlements & Experts 16(4):43 (Apr) 2000

INDOMETHACIN
Femoral Avascular Necrosis

A 33-year-old patient was on chronic indomethacin therapy (150 mg daily for eight months) prior to a laminectomy and discectomy for sciatic pain secondary to a lumbar 4/5 intervertebral disc prolapse. Although the patient was initially pain free, right hip pain recurred approximately four months post surgery. Indomethacin therapy was reinitiated for two months without pain relief. There were no concurrent medications during this time period. At a one year follow-up evaluation, a physical examination revealed flexion restriction and shortening of the affected hip. Radiographic examination revealed collapse of the right femoral head due to avascular necrosis. All other hematological parameters were within normal limits.

The authors concluded that indomethacin was responsible for avascular femoral head necrosis in this patient as a result of chronic dosing. A proposed mechanism of action was that microfractures in weight bearing joints are not allowed to heal during NSAID therapy, predisposing to further breakdown. In addition, indomethacin has been shown to interfere with the production of cartilage matrix in animals. The authors suggested that patients on long term indomethacin should be monitored for early detection of avascular necrosis.

Prathapkumar KR et al. (Flat No 2, HM Stanley Hosp, St Asaph, Denbighshire LL17 ORS; e-mail: rajiprathap@netscapeonline.co.uk) Indomethacin induced avascular necrosis of head of femur. Postgrad Med J 76:574–575 (Sep) 2000

KETOPROFEN (Topical)
Acute Renal Failure (First Report*)

A 62-year-old inpatient, hospitalized for inflammatory arthritis of the ankle experienced increases in serum creatinine and urea (673 umol/L and 38 mmol/L) after five days of therapy with colchicine (1 mg daily) and topical ketoprofen (twice daily). She also had a history of chronic renal failure due to polycystic kidney disease but enjoyed stable renal function for several months prior to this episode. Other concurrent medications included rilmenidine, furosemide, atenolol, amlodipine, enalapril, aspirin, sodium bicarbonate, and simvastatin. Acute renal failure was diagnosed and topical ketoprofen, furosemide and enalapril were discontinued. Ketoprofen levels were 4.17 mg/L at six days after the drug was stopped. Renal function returned to baseline after eight days.

The authors concluded that ketoprofen along with angiotensin converting enzyme inhibitors and diuretics were risk factors for the development of kidney failure. However, they suggested that renal function changes were most likely due to ketoprofen due to high plasma concentrations despite topical application. They suggested that topical NSAIDs should be used with caution in patients with renal dysfunction.

Krummel T et al (Dept Nephrology, Hosp Univ, Strasbourg, France) Acute renal failure induced by topical ketoprofen, Br Med J 320:93 (Jan 8) 2000 (letter)

MELOXICAM
Erythema Multiforme

A 19-year-old patient developed oral discomfort when chewing and maculopapular lesions on her palms and soles approximately eight days after starting meloxicam (15 mg daily) for tendonitis. Initial treatment consisted of erythromycin (500 mg every six hours) for suspected acute streptococcal infection. Despite antimicrobial therapy, the lesions worsened, resulting in eventual hospitalization. Although initial laboratory data revealed an elevated white blood cell count, additional laboratory screenings for infectious etiologies were negative. Erythema multiforme was diagnosed and both meloxicam and erythromycin were discontinued. Treatment with intravenous prednisone (50 mg daily) resulted in improvement.

The authors concluded that meloxicam was most likely responsible for this patient's erythema multiforme.

Nikas SN et al (Dept Internal Med, Med Sch, Univ of Ioannina, Ioannina, Greece) Meloxicam induced erythema multiforme. An J Med 107:532–533 (Nov) 1999

NABUMETONE AND WARFARIN
Anticoagulation Potentiation (First Report*)

A 72-year-old man, previously stabilized on warfarin therapy (34 mg/week) with INRs in therapeutic range (2.0 to 2.1), had an increased INR (3.7) within one week after starting nabumetone therapy (750 mg twice daily). Other chronic medications included digoxin, quinidine, topical nitroglycerin, ranitidine, hyoscyamine, zolpidem and multivitamins. Despite a planned reduction in warfarin dosage the patient developed right knee swelling and pain which was diagnosed as hemarthrosis. Warfarin therapy was discontinued and nabumetone continued. Four days prior to surgical repair of the right knee cartilage, symptoms suggestive of a TIA occurred precipitating the prescribing of clopidrogel while continuing nabumetone. Follow-up at one year revealed that the patient did not have any neurologic events and no further occurrences of hemarthrosis during concurrent therapy.

The authors concluded that increases in INR and hemarthrosis were a result of combined nabumetone and warfarin therapy. Possible mechanisms discussed included warfarin metabolism inhibition and/or protein binding displacement. The authors also recommended that all patients on warfarin therapy should be closely monitored when new therapy is added.

Dennis VC et al. Potentiation of oral anticoagulation and hemarthrosis associated with nabumetone. Pharmacotherapy 20(2):234–239 (Feb) 2000

NONSTEROIDAL ANTI-INFLAMMATORY DRUGS (NSAIDs)
Incidence of Congestive Heart Failure in Elderly

In a matched case control study between 1993 and 1995 at two hospital sites, 365 elderly patients admitted for congestive heart failure (mean age 73.6 yrs) were matched with 658 control admissions (mean age: 75.1 yrs). Of the case patients, 149 were hospitalized for the first time with congestive heart failure and 29.5% had used a nonsteroidal anti-inflammatory drug (NSAID) prior to admission. Specifically, approximately one-fifth had used a nonaspirin NSAID in the week prior to admission (20%) or in the month prior to admission (22%). Nonprophylactic aspirin was used by 10.7% of the cases in the week prior to admission and 12.1% in the month prior to admission. Usage of these agents was 9.2% and 6.6% of the controls, respectively. NSAID use (other than low dose aspirin during the previous week) was associated with a twofold increased risk (odds ratio: 2.1) for the hospitalization due to congestive heart failure. In patients with a history of heart disease, this risk was increased further. First admissions for congestive heart failure were also positively related to the higher doses of NSAID dose and those products with longer half-lives.

The authors concluded that NSAIDs were responsible for approximately 19% of congestive heart failure related hospitalizations. The authors also recommended that NSAIDs should be used with caution in patients with a history of cardiovascular disease.

NSAIDs
Page J & Henry D Consumption of NSAIDs and the development of congestive heart failure in elderly patients. An underrecognized public health problem. Arch Intern Med 160:777–784 (Mar 27) 2000

ROFECOXIB
Acute Renal Failure in Renal Transplant Patient
(First Report*)

A 49-year-old renal transplant patient was hospitalized for suspected acute rejection approximately four weeks after starting rofecoxib (50 mg daily) for degenerative joint disease. Concurrent medications included long term cyclosporine and prednisone (dosages not provided) as immunosuppressive therapy for a renal transplant performed nine years earlier. Serum creatinine, previously stabilized within normal limits (1.3 mg/dL) four weeks earlier, progressively increased to 4.0 mg/dL during rofecoxib therapy. Screenings for proteinuria, urinary sediment and eosinophilia were normal.

Serum creatinine returned to 1.2 mg/dL within three days after rofecoxib was discontinued.

The authors concluded that acute renal failure in this patient was related to administration of the selective COX-2 inhibitor, rofecoxib. They suggested that kidney function in a renal transplant patient depends upon the function of both COX isoforms.

Wolf G et al (Univ Hosp Eppendorf, D—20246 Hamburg, Germany) Acute renal failure associated with rofecoxib. Ann Intern Med 133(5):394 (Sep 5) 2000 (letter)

ANALGESICS-OPIATES
FENTANYL (Transdermal)
Heated Patch Results in Overdose & Death, Legal Action

A 36-year-old man used a fentanyl patch with a heating pad and blanket for back pain due to a back injury. The plaintiff claimed that the fatal drug overdose occurred as a result of increased drug delivery from an inadvertently heated patch. In addition, the plaintiff claimed that information was not provided regarding the dangers of heating the patch. A jury awarded a five million dollar award for loss of earnings and relative emotional distress.

Estate of K. Hophan vs Alsa Corp, Janssen Pharmaceutica, Inc., et al Failure to warn of Duragesic's potential to overdose when patch is heated—death—$5 million Pennsylvania verdict. Medical Malpractice Verdicts, Settlements & Experts 15(12):9 (Dec) 1999

FENTANYL AND RITONAVIR
Interaction: Decreased Fentanyl Clearance,
Increased Half-life

In a double blinded, placebo controlled crossover study, 12 health subjects received either oral ritanovir or placebo for three days. Ritanovir was dosed at 200 mg three times daily the first day, followed by 300 mg three times daily on the second day. On the third morning, the last dose of ritonavir or placebo was given. On day two, intravenous fentanyl (5 mcg/kg) was administered over two minutes. Naloxone (0.1 mg) was also administered prior to and with fentanyl to prevent sedative and respiratory effects typically associated with fentanyl. Eleven subjects completed the study; one patient withdrew as a result of nausea and vomiting. Ritonavir reduced fentanyl clearance by 67% (15.6 to 5.2 mL/min/kg) accompanied by increases in AUC (4.8 to 8.8 ng/mL) and fentanyl half-life (9.4 vs 20.1 hrs). Eight of the 11 patients completing the study reported nausea.

The authors concluded that ritonavir inhibited the metabolism of fentanyl, possibly via the CYP3A4 isoenzyme system. They also suggested that decreases in fentanyl elimination may increase the risks of respiratory depression in patients receiving this combination.

Olkkola KT et al (Dept Anesth, Toolo Hosp, Helsinki Univ Central Hosp, PO Box 266, FIN-00029 HYKS, Finland) Ritonavir's role in reducing fentanyl clearance and prolonging its half-life. Anesthesiology 91:681–685 (Sep) 1999

MEPERIDINE
Hypertensive Crisis

A 70-year-old patient became hypertensive (systolic blood pressure: 235 mmHg) during chemoembolization of a carcinoid tumor with doxorubicin (60 mg) in diatrizoate meglumine (10 mL). Concurrent medications included octreotide, dexamethasone and continuous meperidine infusion (10 mg/hr) administered 1.5 hours prior to the procedure. Despite treatment with intravenous labetalol (5 mg), nitroglycerin paste, and intravenous enalapril (0.625 mg), the patient remained hypertensive, ultimately requiring admission to an intensive care unit. The meperidine infusion was discontinued at this time and intravenous nitroprusside initiated. Blood pressure control was eventually achieved. At 12 hours post hypertensive episode, the serum serotonin and urine 5-hydroxyindoleacetic acid level were significantly elevated (14.84 umol/L and 1311 mg/g of creatinine).

The authors suggested that this patient's hypertensive crisis was related to increased serotonin levels caused by serotonin release post chemoembolization and the inhibition of presynaptic serotonin reuptake by meperidine. They concluded that meperidine administration during malignant carcinoid is a dangerous drug-disease combination.

Balestrero LM et al (Cambridge, MA) Hypertensive crisis following meperidine administration and chemoembolization of a carcinoid tumor. Arch Intern Med 160:2394–2395 (Aug 14/28) 2000 (letter)

MEPERIDINE AND RITONAVIR
Interaction: Decreased Meperidine and Increased Normeperidine Concentrations

In an open-label, crossover, pharmacokinetic study, eight healthy volunteers received a single oral dose of meperidine (50 mg). Two days later they started ritonavir therapy (500 mg twice daily) for 13 days. On day 10 another single dose of meperidine was administered. After ritonavir administration the mean meperidine AUC was decreased by 67% (172.3 vs 522.7 ng.hr/mL) and peak concentrations were also decreased by approximately 40% (51.1 vs 125.8 ng/mL). However time to peak concentration was unaffected (1.2 vs 1.5 hrs). In contrast, mean normeperidine AUC was increased by 47% after concurrent ritonavir administration (361.7 vs 246 ng.hr/mL), as were peak concentrations (38.6 vs 20.6 ng/mL). Time to peak concentration was decreased after ritonavir administration (2.7 vs 4 hrs).

The authors suggested that increased normeperidine concentrations reflect an induction of CYP-mediated metabolism via ritonavir. They proposed that CYP1A2 might be the predominant isoenzyme responsible for meperidine metabolism. Another theory suggests that simultaneous induction/inhibition of the competing metabolic pathways results in an overall net induction effect. Although the risk of increased meperidine side effects during concurrent ritonavir therapy appears low, the risk of normeperidine accumulation may be increased.

Piscitelli SC et al (Clinical Center Pharmacy Dept, Bldg. 10, Room IN257, NIH, Bethesda, MD 20892) The effect of ritonavir on the pharmacokinetics of meperidine and normeperidine. Pharmacotherapy 20(5):549–553 (May) 2000

METHADONE AND RITONAVIR
Interaction: Decreased Methadone Effect

A 51-year-old patient, previously stabilized in a methadone program (90 mg daily) for two years, was hospitalized for withdrawal symptoms, which began approximately 5.5 hours prior to admission. Ritonavir (400 mg twice daily), saquinavir (400 mg twice daily), and stavudine (40 mg twice daily) had recently been started seven days earlier. Other chronic medications included TMP/SMX (160/800 mg every other day), fosinopril (20 mg daily), and cimetidine (400 mg twice daily). Liver function tests were consistent with baseline studies, with the exception of an elevated gamma-glutamyl transferase (191 U/L). Methadone levels at the time of admission were 210 ng/mL. The patient was stabilized on increased methadone doses during hospitalization (100 mg daily) and post discharge (130 mg daily).

The authors suggested that ritonavir was most likely responsible for withdrawal symptoms in this patient as a result of decreased methadone serum levels via hepatic isoenzyme induction. They encouraged clinicians to be aware of this possible interaction and recommended that formal clinical studies be performed.

Geletko SM & Erickson AD. Decreased methadone effect after ritonavir initiation. Pharmacotherapy 20(1):93–94 (Jan) 2000

MORPHINE
Respiratory Arrest, Self-Dosing Pump, Legal Action

Within 24 hours after recovering from back surgery for a ruptured disc, an inpatient experienced respiratory arrest as a result of overdosing via a self-dosing pump. Approximately 81 mg of morphine were administered over a 15-hour period prior to the arrest. During the cardiac resuscitation session, two pieces of essential equipment were missing from the emergency cart (e.g., Ambu bag and back board) resulting in a six-minute delay (via medical record documentation) to proper ventilation. Code blue attendants testified, indicating that there was a 2.5 to three minute delay. Severe brain damage occurred with subsequent death.

L Philpott vs St. Luke's Hosp & Reliable Health Care, Inc. Man suffers respiratory arrest from morphine after back surgery while using self-dosing pump—code blue cart doesn't have Ambu bag and back board on it—brain damage and death—$1.5 million Missouri verdict. Med Malpractice Verdicts, Settlements & Experts 16(6):20–21 (Jun) 2000

ANTICONVULSANTS
CARBAMAZEPINE
Systemic Lupus Erythematosus, Cardiac Tamponade

A 45-year-old patient was hospitalized with dyspnea and chest pain approximately eight months after switching from phenytoin to carbamazepine therapy (no dosages provided). Other symptoms included hypotension (90/60 mmHg), tachycardia (114 beats per minute), tachypnea (26 to 30 breaths per minute), and fever. Serum carbamazepine concentrations were within therapeutic range (7.8 mcg/mL). An echocardiogram revealed pericardial effusions consistent with cardiac tamponade, which was relieved via therapeutic pericardiocentesis (850 mL). Although screenings for bacteriological and viral etiologies were negative, blood serologic testing was positive for antinuclear antibodies (1:320) and antihistone antibodies but negative for double stranded DNA (dsDNA). Recovery was uneventful and phenobarbital was substituted for carbamazepine therapy prior to discharge.

The authors concluded that this patient developed cardiac tamponade related to carbamazepine induced systemic lupus erythematosus (SLE)-like syndrome. The presence of antinuclear and antihistone antibodies without dsDNA was highly suggestive of a drug induced SLE syndrome. Although cardiac tamponade is a rare manifestation of SLE, the authors encouraged clinicians to consider this diagnosis in patients who develop chest pain and dyspnea while taking carbamazepine therapy.

Verna SP et al (Univ Pennsylvania Sch Med, 700 Clinical Research Bldg., 415 Curie Blvd, Philadelphia, PA 19104; e-mail:sunliv@att.net) Carbamazepine induced systemic lupus erythematosus tamponade. Chest 117:597–598 (Feb) 2000

CARBAMAZEPINE
Multiple Sclerosis Worsening

Two cases of multiple sclerosis worsening were described in patients after receiving low dose carbamazepine.

Patient 1: A 48-year-old multiple sclerosis patient developed severe weakness impairing normal walking activity approximately two days after starting oral carbamazepine (100 mg three times daily). Other medications were not provided. However, the patient was able to walk unassisted within two days after stopping carbamazepine. Although the patient was asymptomatic for one week after carbamazepine was restarted at a lower dosage (50 mg three times daily), severe leg weakness recurred after the dosage was increased to previous levels (100 mg three times daily). Once again, symptoms resolved within two days after the drug was stopped.

Patient 2: A 67-year-old multiple sclerosis patient was unable to stand due to severe leg weakness, which began two days after oral carbamazepine (100 mg three times daily) was started for trigeminal neuralgia. Other concurrent medications were not provided. Treatment with intravenous methylprednisolone was unsuccessful (500 mg daily for five days). Two days after carbamazepine was stopped, the patient was able to walk again with a frame.

The authors noted that similar effects were observed in three additional multiple sclerosis patients after carbamazepine therapy (300 to 600 mg daily). Like the cases reported above, symptoms began within three days after drug initiation and reversed after medication withdrawal (within two days). They suggested that carbamazepine may block sodium channels in the demyelinated axonal membrane, interfering with conduction action potential.

Ransaransing G et al (DeKeyser J, Dept Neurol, Acad Zickenhuis Groningen, Hanzeplein 1, 9700 RB Groningen, Netherlands; email:j.h.a.de.keyser@neuro.azg.nl) Worsening of symptoms of multiple sclerosis associated with carbamazepine. Br Med J 320:1113 (Apr 22) 2000 (letter)

DIVALPROEX SODIUM
Hypothermia, Thermoregulatory Dysfunction
(First Reports*)

Five cases of hypothermia or thermoregulatory dysfunction with divalproex sodium were reported.

Patient 1: An 85-year-old patient developed hypothermia (oral temperature: $36°C$) and confusion shortly after starting divalproex sodium (250 mg three times daily). Valproic acid levels were 25 mcg/mL. Despite the use of heating blankets, the patient's body temperature continued to fall ($32.2°C$) with further deterioration in mental status. Divalproex sodium was stopped after 10 days and within eight hours, the patient's body temperature slowly rose to $36.4°C$. Within 12 hours, normal body temperature was achieved and mental status improved.

Patient 2: A 44-year-old patient developed mild lethargy and hypothermia (oral temperatures: $32.2°C$ to $33.9°C$) within 18 months after starting divalproex sodium (250 mg three times daily titrated to 2000 mg daily).

Valproic acid levels were 45 mcg/mL. Immediately after the dose was reduced (250 mg three times daily) the patient's temperature rose by 4°F. Temperature and communications normalization was achieved once the drug was completely discontinued two weeks later.

Patient 3: A 73-year-old patient became confused, drowsy and hypothermic (oral temperatures: 35°C to 35.8°C) within 17 days of starting divalproex sodium (750 mg three times daily) for a bipolar disorder. Concurrent medications included digoxin, gabapentin, apresoline, glipizide, furosemide, ranitidine, colestipol, and aspirin (no dosages provided). Valproic acid levels were 78 mcg/mL. All symptoms reversed within a few days after both gabapentin and valproic acid were discontinued. No recurrences were noted when lithium carbonate therapy was substituted.

Patient 4: An 80-year-old patient developed lethargy and hypothermia (rectal temperatures: 32.5°C and 33.9°C) requiring hospitalization during chronic divalproex sodium therapy (250 mg twice daily for two years) for agitation related to Alzheimer's disease. Despite subtherapeutic valproic acid concentrations (15 to 20 mcg/mL), the drug was effective. Concurrent medications included levothyroxine, digoxin, and furosemide. Symptoms were diagnosed as possibly related to risperidone withdrawal. However, within two days after valproic acid was tapered and stopped, mental status returned to baseline and temperatures rose to 35.6 and 36.9°C. Hypothermia recurred after divalproex sodium was inadvertently restarted five days later.

Patient 5: A 48-year-old patient reported dramatic improvement in heat intolerance after divalproex acid was added (500 mg three times daily) to his anticonvulsant regimen (e.g. phenytoin, carbamazepine, and phenobarbital). His body temperature dropped by one degree Fahrenheit. Once divalproex acid was discontinued because of tremors, heat intolerance returned immediately.

The authors concluded that these were the first reports of hypothermic reactions related to divalproex sodium administration and suggested that they were related to its GABA agonist activities.

Zachariah SB et al. (Neurology Serv (127), Bay Pines VA Med Center, PO Box 5005, Bay Pines, FL 33744; e-mail:sally.zachariah@med.va.gov) Hypothermia and thermoregulatory derangements induced by valproic acid. Neurology 55:150–151 (Jul) 2000

GABAPENTIN
Asterixis

A 60-year-old inpatient developed asterixis in both hands on the fourth day of gabapentin therapy for refractory severe postherpetic neuralgia. Gabapentin was titrated from 300 mg daily on the first day, to twice daily administration on the second day and three times daily on the third day.

Despite pain relief and laboratory values within normal ranges, gabapentin was discontinued. Symptoms resolved within three days after the drug was withdrawn. Rechallenge with gabapentin at a lower dose (300 mg daily) resulted in approximately 50% pain relief without asterixis recurrences.

The authors suggested that gabapentin was the most likely cause of asterixis in this patient, possibly related to enhanced GABAnergic transmission.

Jacob PC et al (Dept Med (Neurology), College of Med, PO Box 35, Sultan Qaboos Univ, 123 Muscat, Oman) Asterixis induced by gabapentin. Clin Neuropharmacol 23: 53 (Feb) 2000

GABAPENTIN AND PROPRANOLOL
Dystonia

A 68-year-old patient developed paroxysmal dystonia in both hands approximately two days after propranolol (80 mg daily) was added to gabapentin therapy (900 mg daily) for essential tremor. Although previous unsuccessful therapy included primidone and clonazepam, no other concurrent medications were provided. Dystonic episodes lasted approximately one minute. Other neurological testing, laboratory values, electrolytes and hormonal levels, however, were within normal ranges. The abnormal movements rapidly resolved after the propranolol dosage was reduced (40 mg daily). Combined gabapentin and propranolol therapy was uneventful.

The authors suggested that a synergistic effect occurred between propranolol and gabapentin therapy causing abnormal movements. They proposed that propranolol may have stimulated gabapentin modulation pathways.

Palomeras E et al (Unit Neurologia, Hosp de Mataro, Carratera Cirera, s/n 08304, Mataro, Spain; email: neurologia2@csm.scs.es) Dystonia in a patient treated with propranolol and gabapentin. Arch Neurol 57:570–571 (Apr) 2000

LAMOTRIGINE
Hypersensitivity, Disseminated Intravascular Coagulation

A 27-year-old woman was hospitalized with fever, headache, myalgia, neck pain and nuchal rigidity approximately seven days after starting lamotrigine therapy for seizures. The only other medication taken was phenobarbital (no dosage provided). Abnormal laboratory parameters included white blood cell count (2,500/mm^3), and platelets (94,000/mm^3). While hospitalized her condition progressively worsened, developing a generalized macular rash and trunk. Abnormal lab values at this time included AST (348 U/L), lactate dehydrogenase (2,666 U/L), creatine phosphokinase (133 IU/L), prothrombin time (13.2 seconds) and partial thromboplastin time (36.2 seconds) The patient was diagnosed as having a hypersensitivity reaction with disseminated intravascular coagulation. Lamotrigine was stopped at this time, resulting in gradual improvement over the next four days and a complete recovery by eight days.

The authors concluded that this patient experienced a hypersensitivity reaction to lamotrigine possibly caused by toxic drug metabolites (arene oxide products) via cytochrome P450 metabolism.

Sarris BM & Wong JG (Yale Univ Sch Med, Waterbury Hosp Health Center, 64 Robbins St, Waterbury, CT 06721) Multisystem hypersensitivity reaction to lamotrigine. Neurology 53:1367 (Oct) 1999 (letter)

LAMOTRIGINE
Agranulocytosis (First Report*)

Neutropenia and agranulocytosis were discovered during a hospitalization of a 30-year psychiatric patient, two weeks after valproic acid (slow titration up to 250 mg at bedtime) was added to lamotrigine therapy (100 mg daily). Other concurrent medications also included clonazepam (2 mg twice daily), sustained release bupropion (150 mg twice daily), and olanzapine (5 mg nightly as needed). The white blood cell count was 3,200 and absolute neutrophil count was 446, which both changed to 2,600 and 580, respectively within two days. Leukopenia resolved after lamotrigine was discontinued and did not recur while the patient was continued on valproic acid therapy (750 mg nightly).

The authors suggested that an interaction among lamotrigine, valproic acid and possibly, olanzapine may have lowered the threshold for lamotrigine induced agranulocytosis.

Solvason HB (Stanford CA) Agranulocytosis associated with lamotrigine. Am J Psychiatry 157(10):1704 (Oct) 2000 (letter)

LAMOTRIGINE
Photosensitivity Rash

Two cases of photosensitivity rashes are described in patients taking lamotrigine therapy for longer than three months.

Patient 1: A 42-year-old man developed an acute maculopapular rash with pruritis approximately 24 hours after significant sun exposure. Chronic medications included lamotrigine (100 mg twice daily) and haloperidol (20 mg twice daily) for a bipolar type schizoaffective disorder. No information was provided regarding treatment or symptom resolution.

Patient 2: A 30-year-old woman developed an acute maculopapular rash with itching within one day after sun exposure in a solarium. Chronic medications included lamotrigine (100 mg twice daily). Although the rash resolved after lamotrigine was stopped, the time required for the disappearance of symptoms was not provided.

The authors concluded that lamotrigine was responsible for photosensitive rashes in both patients and recommended that patients taking lamotrigine should avoid prolonged sunlight exposure. A mechanism of action was not provided.

Bozikas V et al (Thessaloniki, Greece) Lamotrigine induced rash after sun exposure. Am J Psychiatry 156:2015–2016 (Dec) 1999 (letter)

PHENYTOIN
Fatal Hypersensitivity Syndrome

An 85-year-old woman was hospitalized after a syncopal episode accompanied by fever, rigors and pruritic rash. Medications included metformin (500 mg twice daily), tolbutamide (500 mg twice daily), nifedipine (10 mg twice daily), risperidone (1 mg daily) and phenytoin (300 mg nightly), which was added one month prior to admission. Elevated laboratory values included serum eosinophils (0.7×10^9/L), creatinine (192 umol/L), alanine and aspartate transaminases (415 and 202 IU), alkaline phosphatase (275 IU/L), bilirubin (25 umol/L), and C-reactive protein (103 mg/L). Treatment included empiric antibiotics, corticosteroids and antihistamines. All medications except phenytoin were stopped on hospital day three and phenytoin was stopped on hospital day seven. The patient's condition progressively deteriorated, developing cardiac, renal and hepatic failure, resulting in death 12 days after admission. Autopsy revealed enlarged lungs, liver, and spleen. Histological examination of the heart revealed eosinophils infiltration without necrosis or fibrosis. Skin biopsy revealed toxic epidermal necrolysis.

The authors concluded that phenytoin hypersensitivity syndrome was responsible for this patient's death. The exact mechanism of action is not clear but may be related to the development of immune complexes, delayed hypersensitivity allergies, altered lymphocyte function or toxic metabolite production.

Mahadeva U et al (Leen E: Histopathology Lab, James Connolly Mem Hosp, Blanchardstown, Dublin 15, Ireland) Fatal phenytoin hypersensitivity syndrome. Postgrad Med J 75:734–736 (Dec) 1999

PHENYTOIN, VALPROATE
Intravenous Site Reactions

In a retrospective chart review of two double blind, randomized clinical trial data, the incidences of intravenous site reactions were collected in neurotrauma patients receiving either intravenous phenytoin or valproate. In the first study, 210 patients (mean age: 34 yrs) received intravenous phenytoin in maintenance doses ranging from 100 to 600 mg. In the second study,

255 patients (mean age: 37 yrs) received intravenous valproate in doses ranging from 150 to 1000 mg and 130 patients (mean age: 35 yrs) received maintenance doses ranging from 200 to 550 mg. Intravenous site reactions occurred in 18% of the valproate group and in 25% of the phenytoin group. Although the drugs were administered via central or peripheral routes, all reactions occurred with the peripheral route. When central line administration patients were excluded, the incidence rate rose to 21% and 30%, respectively.

The authors concluded that both phenytoin and valproate cause intravenous site reactions. Loading doses were responsible for most events.

Anderson GD et al (Dept Pharmacy, Box 357630, Univ Washington, Seattle WA 98195; e-mail:gaila@u.washington.edu) Incidence of intravenous site reactions in neurotrauma patients receiving valproate or phenytoin. Ann Pharmacother 34:697–702 (Jun) 2000

VALPROATE
Hyperandrogenism, Polycystic Ovaries

Three cases of drug induced reproductive endocrine disorders were described in women taking valproate for seizures.

Patient 1: A 34-year-old patient gradually gained 52 kg during valproate therapy for seizures over a 17 year period. She also developed secondary amenorrhea with high serum testosterone levels (11.2 nmol/L), both of which responded to progestin therapy. Because these effects were diagnosed as possibly related to valproate therapy, lamotrigine therapy was substituted at an initial dose of 200 mg daily and gradually increased to 600 mg daily. During the first year of lamotrigine therapy, the patient lost 17 kg and developed regular menstruation cycles. In addition, serum testosterone levels decreased from 3.5 nmol/L to 2.5 nmol/L, and polycystic ovary changes initially visualized on ultrasound during valproate therapy reversed after lamotrigine was started.

Patient 2: A 21-year-old patient gradually gained 13.5 kg during valproate therapy for seizures over a two year period. She also developed secondary amenorrhea with hyperprolactinemia and high serum testosterone levels (5.5 nmol/L). Pelvic ultrasound revealed subcapsular ovarian cysts. Treatment with bromocriptine resulted in normalization of serum prolactin levels but hyperandrogenism and amenorrhea persisted. Because these effects were diagnosed as possibly related to valproate therapy, lamotrigine therapy was substituted (200 mg daily). During the first year of lamotrigine therapy, the patient lost 10 kg and developed random menstruation cycles (4 per year). In addition, serum testosterone levels decreased from 4.5 nmol/L to 1.6 nmol/L. However, polycystic ovary changes initially visualized on ultrasound remained the same.

Patient 3: A 31-year-old patient maintained her weight during valproate therapy (600 mg daily) for seizures over a four year period. After two years of therapy, her menstrual cycles were regular, but she had high serum testosterone levels (7.5 nmol/L). Pelvic ultrasound revealed normal ovaries at this time. After four years of valproate therapy, menstrual cycles were still regular and serum testosterone levels had decreased (2.5 nmol/L), but ultrasound revealed changes consistent with polycystic ovaries. After lamotrigine substitution (titration to maintenance dose: 500 mg daily) for valproate, no changes in weight occurred during the first year of therapy. However, serum testosterone decreased from 2.5 nmol/L to 1.8 nmol/L and polycystic ovary changes reversed. Menstrual cycles also remained regular.

The authors concluded that the development of reproductive endocrine disorders in these women was related to valproate therapy. They suggested that the drug-induced weight gain accompanied by hyperinsulinemia may be related to the development of hyperandrogenism and polycystic ovary changes, or that valproate may have a direct action on serum testosterone levels. The authors recommended that further investigations should be performed in this area to confirm a relationship between valproate and hyperandrogenism and polycystic ovary changes.

Isojarvi JIY & Tapanainen JS (Dept Neurology, Univ Oulu, FIN-90220, Oulu, Finland; e-mail:jouko@isojarvi@oulu.fi) Valproate, hyperandrogenism, and polycystic ovaries: A report of 3 cases. Arch Neurol 57:1064–1068 (Jul) 2000

VALPROIC ACID
Fatal Pulmonary Hemorrhage

A 30-year-old patient was hospitalized with fever, cough, and dyspnea. She had been stabilized on valproic acid therapy for approximately 10 years. Additional symptoms three weeks prior to admission included bruising on the upper and lower limbs when the patient sought medical attention for a viral nasal-pharyngeal infection. Chest x-ray upon admission revealed lower lobe infiltrates. Abnormal lab values included white blood cell count (3000/uL), platelets (15,000/uL), and hemoglobin (4.9 g/dL). Serum valproate levels upon admission were elevated (124 mcg/mL). Treatment included broad-spectrum antibiotics and red blood cell and platelet transfusions. Cytological examination of lavage fluid indicated alveolar hemorrhage. On hospital day three the patient's condition worsened, suffering a cardiopulmonary failure with subsequent death.

The authors noted that this was the first report of fatal pulmonary hemorrhage associated with valproate monotherapy. They suggested that the initial viral infection may have precipitated thrombocytopenia. They also cautioned clinicians to monitor platelet function in patients on long term valproate therapy who develop bruising or viral infections.

Sleiman C et al (Centre Hosp de Chartres, Ser de Pneumologie, BP 407, 28000 Chartres, France) Fatal pulmonary hemorrhage during high dose valproate monotherapy. Chest 117:613 (Feb) 2000 (letter)

VALPROIC ACID, VALPROATE SODIUM, DIVALPROEX SODIUM
Pancreatitis, FDA Advisory

On July 31, 2000, the FDA and manufacturer (Abbott Laboratories) of valproic acid and its derivatives (e.g., divalproex sodium and valproate sodium) notified health professionals regarding new labeling changes in the product insert. Specifically, a boxed warning has been revised regarding the potential for the development of life threatening pancreatitis. Cases have been reported in both children and adults and the onset of symptoms has occurred soon after the initiation of therapy and as late as several years of therapy. Although pancreatitis has been listed as a potential adverse event associated with valproic acid (and derivatives) therapy, it is now listed in a black box warning. It should be noted that these recent changes have been based on FDA discussions with the manufacturer, and are not based on an increased reporting rate of pancreatitis. Some of the cases have been described as hemorrhagic with rapid progression of symptoms, including eventual death. Patients should be counseled regarding symptoms suggestive of pancreatitis, including abdominal pain, vomiting, and/or anorexia and instructed to seek medical attention if these events occur.

New product labeling for valproic acid and derivatives. (Jul) 2000. http://www.fda.gov/med-watch/safety/2000/depako.pd

VALPROIC ACID
Pancreatitis

A 37-year-old schizophrenic patient sought medical attention for epigastric pain, fever, and vomiting approximately 17 months after starting valproic acid therapy (1 gram twice daily). Concurrent medications included phenobarbital (200 mg daily), trazodone (200 mg daily), thiothixene (20 mg daily), propranolol (40 mg three times daily) and benztropine (2 mg daily). Symptoms worsened to include confusion, disorientation and ataxia and the patient was eventually admitted with increased abdominal girth. Abnormal laboratory values upon admission included elevated amylase (91 IU/L), lipase (58 IU/dL), serum alkaline phosphatase (139 IU/L), and gamma-glutamyltransferase (163 IU/L). Valproic acid was discontinued during the hospital stay. An abdominal CT scan confirmed pancreatitis possibly induced by valproic acid.

Rechallenge with valproic acid (1 gram twice daily) 19 months later resulted in severe stomach and joint pain almost two months after starting therapy. At this time concurrent medications included phenobarbital (200 mg daily), thioridazine (50 mg at bedtime), long acting propranolol

(120 mg twice daily), hydrocodone/acetaminophen (5 mg/500 mg), ibuprofen, hydroxyzine, temazepam and magnesium hydroxide. Lipase and amylase levels were elevated (101 IU/dL and 275 IU/L). Recurrent pancreatitis was diagnosed and after supportive treatment the patient was eventually discharged.

The authors concluded that this patient developed recurrent pancreatitis as a result of valproic acid therapy. They also observed that although several other medications were taken, none had been previously associated as direct causative agents of pancreatitis.

Fecik SE et al (VA Med Center, San Diego, CA 92161) Recurrent acute pancreatitis associated with valproic acid use for mood stabilization. J Clin Psychopharmacol 19(5): 483–484 (Oct) 1999 (letter)

VIGABATRIN
Visual Loss

A total of 13 adult patients (mean age: 42 yrs) were withdrawn from a larger cohort study of 39 patients receiving vigabatrin for refractory seizures. Vigabatrin was discontinued because of a lack of efficacy or visual loss possibly related to drug administration. The mean dose during the study was 5.581 grams daily for 31 to 78 months (median 55.5 months). Re-evaluation of these patients for long term follow-up occurred at a mean of 161 days (range: 87 to 314 days) after vigabatrin was stopped. During vigabatrin therapy, 70% of the patients had visual field constrictions of 10 to 20 degrees in at least one eye and 70% had mean static field defects greater than 3 dB. Field constrictions persisted in 69% (9/13) of the patients, and sensitivity loss across the retina persisted in half (6/12). During vigabatrin therapy, 92% of the patients had reductions in amplitudes of oscillatory potentials and flicker ERG, 62% had reductions in cone ERG, and 38% had reductions in rod ERG. Although none of these variables improved overall, some individuals had bilateral improvements. During therapy 54% of the patients experienced reduced visual acuity and 31% had mild reductions in color vision, which persisted as a group at re-evaluation post-therapy. There was no relationship between these parameters and total dose or duration of therapy. However, the three patients who experienced the greatest improvements were among the youngest in the group (ages: 22, 29, and 31) and had received lower doses.

The authors concluded that overall visual losses associated with vigabatrin did not appear to improve in the group, but a few individuals experienced improvements in ERG amplitudes.

Johnson MA et al (419 W Redwood St, Suite 420, Baltimore, MD 21201-1734) Visual loss from vigabatrin. Effect of stopping the drug. Neurology 55:40–45 (Jul) 2000

ANTIDEPRESSANTS
AMITRIPTYLINE
Cardiac Abnormalities Mimicking Acute Infarction

A 44-year-old patient was hospitalized after an amitriptyline overdose with dilated pupils and metabolic acidosis. Upon admission serum electrolytes were normal. The patient was intubated with mechanical ventilation. Immediate treatment included gastric lavage and activated charcoal. Serum amitriptyline levels upon admission were 4880 ng/mL but decreased to 1310 ng/mL after 16 hours. Electrocardiograms performed upon admission revealed sinus tachycardia (125 beats/min) with QRS interval widening and QT interval prolongation. However, after 16 hours, repeat cardiograms revealed ST elevation and T wave conversion indicating an anteroseptal subepicardial injury. This unusual presentation on cardiogram lasted for four days. The QT interval normalized after three days. The patient recovered within 10 days and was discharged.

The authors noted that electrocardiogram changes, such as QT and QRS prolongation are expected in tricyclic antidepressant overdoses. However, cardiac changes mimicking acute infarction are not usual.

Zakanthinos E et al (ICU, Evangelismos Hosp, Ipsilantou St, 4S 47, 10675, Athens, Greece) Abnormal atrial and ventricular repolarization resembling myocardial injury after tricyclic antidepressant drug intoxication. Heart 83:353–354 (Mar) 2000

AMITRIPTYLINE
Munchausen Syndrome by Proxy,
Cardiac Arrhythmias, Seizures

A five-year-old patient was hospitalized with general seizures and polymorphic ventricular tachycardia, which progressed to ventricular fibrillation. Although laboratory values were within normal ranges, ECG displayed a prolonged QTc interval. Treatment included intravenous diazepam, defibrillation and a lidocaine infusion (dosages not provided). The patient remained drowsy for two days while hospitalized but eventually improved and was discharged. Although no medications were taken prior to the hospitalization, the patient was discharged on propranolol, amiodarone and sodium valproate for an idiopathic ventricular tachycardia and seizure disorder. He was rehospitalized two months later in cardiac arrest. An ECG during this hospitalization also revealed arrhythmias. Because of hyperactive behavior alternating with drowsiness, a toxicological screening was performed and revealed high concentrations of tricyclic antidepressants (898 nmol/L). Suspected Munchausen syndrome by proxy was confirmed by the child's history of the mother giving him yellow tablets daily (later identified as amitriptyline 50 mg). A repeated tricyclic antidepressant level performed four days later, revealed a reduced concentration of 429 nmol/L.

The authors concluded that this child experienced amitriptyline induced cardiac arrhythmias and seizures as a result of chronic amitriptyline overdosing.

Manikoth P et al (Dept Pediatrics, Royal Hosp, PO Box 1331, PC 111, Seeb, Sultanate of Oman) A child with cardiac arrhythmia and convulsions. Lancet 354:2046 (Dec 11) 1999 (letter)

AMITRIPTYLINE
Hypersensitivity Reaction (First Report*)

A 24-year-old woman was hospitalized with a morbilliform rash approximately three weeks after starting amitriptyline therapy for depression (25 mg twice daily). Other symptoms upon admission included fever, pruritus, anxiety, tachycardia (125 beats/min) and mild scaling. A blood count revealed increased eosinophils (25%). Serum aspartate aminotransferase and alanine aminotransferase were also elevated (87 U/L and 103 U/L, respectively). Serological testing for infectious etiologies was negative. Skin biopsy revealed a moderate eosinophilic infiltration consistent with a drug eruption. After amitriptyline was stopped and intravenous prednisolone (25 mg daily) was administered for two weeks, the rash began improving. The patient became afebrile within five days after the amitriptyline was stopped. At a one-month follow-up evaluation, skin and blood tests were within normal limits.

The authors concluded that amitriptyline induced a hypersensitivity reaction in this patient. They also noted that this is the first report of such a case and cautioned clinicians regarding this potential risk.

Milionis HJ et al (Dept Internal Med, Med Sch, Univ Ioannina, GR 451 10 Ioannina, Greece) Hypersensitivity syndrome caused by amitriptyline administration.

BUPROPION
Overdose: Cardiotoxicity

A 16-year-old girl was admitted to the emergency room for seizures induced from an overdose of bupropion (15 of the 100 mg sustained release tablets). Upon admission, the initial physical examination revealed tachypnea with a decreased respiratory rate (18 breaths/min). Postictally, the patient remained combative with slurred speech. An electrocardiogram, however, revealed an increased ventricular rate (150 beats/min) and a prolonged QTc interval (600 msec). Treatment included adenosine, which was unsuccessful in reversing ventricular tachycardia and activated charcoal to blunt absorption. Despite these attempts the patient continued to have seizures, which were controlled with anticonvulsants. Agitation and dysarthrias resolved within 12 hours after admission and cardiac abnormalities reversed at a slower rate but completely resolved without treatment. The authors noted that cardiac conduction delays and neurotoxicity were caused by a low dose bupropion overdose in this patient. They suggested early treatment and close cardiac monitoring for all bupropion overdoses.

Shrier M et al (Dept Pediatrics, Univ Med & Dentistry of NJ, Robert Wood Johnson Med Sch at Camden, Camden, NJ) Cardiotoxicity associated with bupropion overdose. Ann Emergency Med 35:100 (Jan) 2000 (letter)

FLUOXETINE
Precipitation of Pheochromocytoma (First Report*)

A 29-year-old patient developed palpitations, nausea headache, sweating and headache approximately a few days after a fluoxetine dosage increase from 20 mg to 40 mg daily. Upon hospital admission, the patient was agitated and anxious with fluctuating hyper/hypotensive episodes (250/140 and 80/30 mmHg). Elevated 24 hour levels of noradrenaline (10.3 nmol/day), adrenaline (32 nmol/day) and vanillylmandelic acid (134 umol/day) were indicative of pheochromocytoma. Surgical removal of the right adrenal gland was performed after magnetic resonance imaging revealed a mass. Histological examination validated the pheochromocytoma diagnosis. Follow-up was uneventful.

The authors suggested that fluoxetine inhibition of serotonin reuptake increased serotonin levels, which may have increased the sensitivity of noradrenaline receptors. These effects precipitated hemodynamic abnormalities, which unmasked a silent pheochromocytoma.

Kashyap AS (3-B Wanowrie Rd, Pune 411040, India) Phaeochromocytoma unearthed by fluoxetine. Postgrad Med J 76:303 (May) 2000 Postgrad Med J 76:361–363 (Jun) 2000

FLUOXETINE AND BUSPIRONE
Serotonin Syndrome (First Report*)

A 37-year-old patient became confused, uncoordinated, had difficulty with thought organization, and developed spasms within four weeks after adding buspirone to fluoxetine (20 mg daily) for refractory generalized anxiety. Buspirone was initiated at 5 mg twice daily and titrated to 30 mg twice daily. The patient had been taking the full dose for only four days when symptoms developed. Additional symptoms included extensive sweating and diarrhea and were most severe in the morning within two to four hours after drug administration. The patient reported that symptoms resolved within two days after the buspirone was discontinued. At follow-up one week later the patient was asymptomatic.

The author suggested that combination therapy with buspirone and fluoxetine caused serotonin syndrome in this patient. Close monitoring of patients on this combination was recommended.

Manos GH (Dept Psychiatry, Naval Med Center—Portsmouth, Portsmouth, VA 23708; e-mail:ghmanos@iname.com) Possible serotonin syndrome associated with buspirone added to fluoxetine. Ann Pharmacotherapy 34:871–874 (Jul/Aug) 2000

MILNACIPRAN
Raynaud's Syndrome

A 35-year-old woman developed Raynaud's syndrome in the index fingers approximately two months after starting milnacipran (100 mg daily) for depression. Other chronic medications included zopiclone and prazepam (no dosages provided). The patient had a similar reaction to beta-blockers three years prior to this event. Upon further examination, a capillarioscopy revealed hypoperfusion but the number of vascular loops were normal although not very discernible. Symptoms resolved within one week after milnacipran was discontinued.

The authors concluded that milnacipran was responsible for Raynaud's syndrome in this patient possibly related to vasospasm induced by serotonin-reuptake inhibition.

Bourgade B et al (A. Jonville-Bera, Dept Clin Pharmacol, Hopital Bretonneau, 2 boulevard Tonnelle, Tours, Cedex 37044, France; e-mail:jonville-bera@ chu.med.univ-tours.fr) Raynaud's syndrome in a patient treated with milnacipran. Ann Pharmacotherapy 33: 1009–1010 (Sep) 1999 (letter)

NEFAZODONE AND TRAZODONE
Interaction: Serotonin Syndrome (First Report*)

A 60-year-old patient developed serotonin syndrome after three days of combined therapy with trazodone (25 to 50 mg daily) added to nefazodone (500 mg daily). Initial symptoms included hypertension (240/120 mmHg) which required an emergency room visit. Other symptoms included intermittent numbness of the face and right hand, temporary rash, nausea, loose stools, difficulty concentrating and confusion. A physical examination revealed restlessness, hyperreflexia, dilated pupils and sweating. Abnormal laboratory values included increased creatinine kinase levels (180 U/L) and total cholesterol (249.8 mg/dL). Both medications were discontinued. Treatment included labetalol, clonidine, amlodipine, and irbesartan. Hypertension resolved within 48 hours and all other symptoms resolved within 12 hours.

The authors concluded that this patient developed serotonin syndrome as a result of combined nefazodone and trazodone therapy. They noted that this is the first case report associated with this combined therapy.

Margolese HC & Chouinard G (Montreal Que, Canada) Serotonin syndrome from addition of low-dose trazodone to nefazodone. Am J Psychiatry 157(6):1022 (Jun) 2000

PAROXETINE
Hyponatremia

A 97-year-old man was hospitalized for progressive lethargy, confusion, weakness and stupor approximately four days after starting paroxetine therapy (20 mg daily) for depression. The only other chronic medication was aspirin (100 mg daily). Although a physical examination revealed no obvious abnormalities, decreased laboratory values included serum sodium (104 mmol/L) and urine sodium (30 mmol/L). Other tests were within normal ranges, including thyroid function, ACTH rapid stimulation test, albumin, liver function tests and other routine biochemical tests. After SIADH (syndrome of inappropriate secretion of antidiuretic hormone) was diagnosed, paroxetine was discontinued, and treatment with 3% sodium chloride infusion was initiated (0.5 mL/min). Within 24 hours, the patient's condition improved and the serum sodium concentration normalized by hospital day five. Recovery was uneventful and the patient was eventually discharged without further recurrences of hyponatremia during follow-up.

The authors concluded that paroxetine was responsible for hyponatremia in this patient. A mechanism of action for this adverse event is not clearly established.

Odeh M et al (PO Box 6477, Haifa 31063, Israel) Severe life-threatening hyponatremia during paroxetine therapy. J Clin Pharmacol 39:1290–1291 (Nov) 1999

PAROXETINE, SERTRALINE
Mydriasis

Three cases of mydriasis are described in young patients during short-term selective serotonin reuptake inhibitor therapy.

Patient 1: A nine-year-old patient developed dilated pupils (6 mm) which were reactive to direct light, approximately five days after starting paroxetine (10 mg daily). Symptoms resolved upon paroxetine withdrawal but returned when the drug was restarted at a lower dose (5 mg daily). Symptoms reversed again when the drug was discontinued.

Patient 2: An 11-year-old patient developed dilated pupils (8 mm) which were poorly reactive to light, approximately one week after starting sertraline therapy for major depression (50 mg daily for five days then 100 mg daily). Symptoms abated but persisted one month after the sertraline dosage was reduced (50 mg daily). The drug was eventually discontinued.

Patient 3: A 14-year-old patient developed dilated pupils (8 mm) which were reactive to direct light within one month after sertraline was added to his regimen (50 mg daily for five days, then 100 mg daily). Concurrent medications included valproic acid (500 mg twice daily). Mydriasis eventually resolved with continued sertraline therapy for two months. The authors concluded that selective serotonin reuptake inhibitors were most likely the cause of mydriasis in these young patients. They proposed that the rapid dosage increase within five days may have precipitated the adverse event and that children and adolescents, like those over 50 years of age, may be at higher risk for this side effect. Clinicians were encouraged to consider this effect when patients on selective serotonin reuptake inhibitors present with dilated pupils.

Larson M & Folstein S (Tufts Univ, Boston, MA) Selective serotonin reuptake inhibitor induced mydriasis. J Am Acad Child Adolesc Psychiatry 39(2):138–139 (Feb) 2000

PAROXETINE AND RISPERIDONE
Serotonin Syndrome (First Report*)

A 53-year-old patient with depression developed abnormal mouth and leg jerking movements approximately nine weeks after being switched to risperidone (3 mg daily) and paroxetine (20 mg daily). Previous unsuccessful medications included nortriptyline (100 mg at night), haloperidol (15 mg at night) and benztropine (1 mg twice daily). One week after the patient stopped the medications he became confused, disorganized and apathetic. Paroxetine and risperidone were restarted at twice the previous dosages (40 mg and 6 mg daily, respectively). Within a few hours after restarting the medications, he developed ataxia, tremors, shivering with reappearance of bilateral jerking movements. Physical examination at the emergency room revealed hypertension, tachycardia, and difficulty in arousal. Additional symptoms included disorientation, visual hallucinations, and hyperreflexia without rigidity. Within two days after risperidone and paroxetine were discontinued, confusion reversed and nortriptyline was substituted (titrated up to 100 mg nightly) without event. Post discharge oral haloperidol (10 mg twice daily) and diphenhydramine (50 mg nightly) were added to his regimen. At follow-up nine months later the patient was symptom free without depression.

The authors concluded that this was the first case report of serotonin syndrome related to concurrent paroxetine and risperidone therapy. One suggested mechanism was hyperserotonism due to increased risperidone levels as both drugs are metabolized by the same cytochrome isoenzyme system. The authors recommended that clinicians be aware of this potential complication with this combination therapy.

Hamilton S & Malone K (NY State Psychiatric Instit & Columbia Univ, Dept Psychiatry, NY, NY 10032) Serotonin syndrome during treatment with paroxetine and risperidone. J Clin Psychopharmacol 29:103–104 (Feb) 2000 (letter) (letter)

REBOXETINE
Hyponatremia

A 72-year-old inpatient hospitalized for stroke rehabilitation developed malaise and nausea approximately eight days after reboxetine therapy was started for depression (4 mg daily). Other medications included aspirin (100 mg daily), enalapril (20 mg daily), and glyburide (5 mg daily). Serum sodium concentrations were 133 mmol/L and 126 mmol/L on the first and fifth days of reboxetine therapy and further decreased to 118 mmol/L after eight days of therapy. Urine sodium concentrations were 181 mmol/L. Urine and serum osmolalities were 430 mOsm/kg and 266 mOsm/kg, respectively. Within six days after reboxetine was discontinued, symptoms reversed and serum sodium concentrations normalized. Rechallenge with reboxetine for six days of therapy resulted in recurrence of nausea, asthenia and hyponatremia by day six. Again, symptoms and hyponatremia reversed when the drug was discontinued.

The authors concluded that reboxetine was responsible for hyponatremia in this patient based on the temporal relationship between the drug initiation and symptom onset. They suggested that hyponatremia was caused by inappropriate secretion of antidiuretic hormone. They also encouraged clinicians to monitor serum sodium in elderly patients who are taking this medication.

Ranieri P et al (P. Richiedei Hosp, 25064 Gusago, Italy) Reboxetine and hyponatremia. N Engl J Med 342:215–216 (Jan 20) 2000 (letter)

SELECTIVE SEROTONIN REUPTAKE INHIBITORS
Upper Gastric Bleeding: Increased Risk

In a population based case-control study, 1899 cases of upper gastrointestinal bleeding or ulcer perforation in older adults (age range: 40 to 79 years) taking selective serotonin reuptake inhibitors (SSRIs) were identified and matched with 10,000 controls. Patient case profiles were reviewed for the use of SSRIs, other antidepressants and/or NSAIDs. Approximately 3.1 (52/1651) of the patients with upper gastrointestinal bleeding were current users of SSRIs. With the exception of fluvoxamine, all SSRIs were associated with an increased risk of upper gastrointestinal bleeding. Relative risk ratios were highest for trazodone (8.6), paroxetine (4.3), and sertraline (3.9). Fluoxetine and clomipramine had similar risk ratios (2.5 and 2.1, respectively). Dosage and duration of therapy were not associated with increased risks. However, the concurrent use of SSRIs with NSAIDs significantly increased the risk of gastrointestinal bleeding when compared to the use of either drug alone (15.6 vs 3.7 vs 2.6).

The authors concluded that most SSRIs increase the risk of upper gastrointestinal bleeding three fold and that this risk is increased when taken in combination with NSAIDs. The authors suggested that a possible depletion of serotonin from platelets might impair a hemostatic response to vascular injury.

De Abajo FJ et al (Div Farmacoepidemiolgia y Farmacovigiliancia Agencia Espanola del Medicamento, 28220 Majadahonda, Madrid Spain) Association between selective serotonin reuptake inhibitors and upper gastrointestinal bleeding: population based case control study. Br Med J 319:1106–1109 (Oct 23) 1999

VENLAFAXINE
Bruxism (First Report*)

A 50-year-old man developed symptoms of bruxism (e.g., jaw clenching and teeth grinding) during the day and night a few days after the addition of oral venlafaxine to his regimen (37.5 mg to 75 mg twice daily). Concurrent medications included valproic acid (1500 mg daily), clonazepam (0.5 mg as needed) and omeprazole (20 mg daily). Oral gabapentin was initiated (300 mg nightly) for the accompanying insomnia and anxiety and all symptoms resolved within two days after starting gabapentin. Venlafaxine therapy was continued without further event.

The authors concluded that bruxism has been reported with other psychotropic medications but this was the first published case report associated with venlafaxine. They suggested that serotonin reuptake inhibition may have a role in the development of these symptoms. They suggested that larger controlled studies are needed to evaluate this potential relationship and the use of gabapentin to reverse symptoms.

Brown ES & Hong SC (Dept Psychiatry, Univ Texas Southwestern Med Center, St. Paul Prof Bldg 1, Ste 600, 5959 Henry Hines Blvd, Dallas, TX 75235-9101) Antidepressant induced bruxism successfully treated with gabapentin. J Am Dental Assoc 130: 1467–1469 (Oct) 1999

VENLAFAXINE AND TRIFLUOPERAZINE
Interaction: Neuroleptic Malignant Syndrome
(First Report*)

A 44-year-old patient with depression was hospitalized for anxiety, malaise and profuse sweating which developed within 12 hours after taking the first dose of venlafaxine (75 mg once daily). The only other chronic medication was trifluoperazine (1 mg three times daily for 10 years). Additional symptoms included tremors, rigidity, hypertension (up to 165/100 mmHg), tachycardia (163 beats per minute) and fever, all indicative of neuroleptic malignant syndrome. Most laboratory parameters were within normal limits with the exception of an elevated creatine phosphokinase (11,320 IU/L) and white blood cell count (23.5×10^9/L). Treatment included dantrolene (70 mg once) and bromocriptine (15 mg twice daily for 48 hrs). Symptoms resolved within 24 hours after psychotropic drugs were discontinued and treatment was initiated. Trifluoperazine was restarted without event during follow-up.

The authors suggested that dopamine inhibition may have been enhanced by adding venlafaxine to existent trifluoperazine therapy, resulting in neuroleptic malignant syndrome.

Nimmagadda SR et al (Acute Psychiatric Assessment Unit, Millview Court, Castle Hill Hosp, Cottingham, Hull, UK; e-mail:seshagiri25@hotmail.com)

Neuroleptic malignant syndrome after venlafaxine. Lancet 354:289–290 (Jan 22) 2000 (letter)

VENLAFAXINE, AMITRIPTYLINE
Serotonin Syndrome

A 75-year-old psychiatric inpatient became confused approximately two weeks after starting venlafaxine for depression. Previous unsuccessful therapy included sertraline (100 mg daily), which was discontinued for lack of effect after 11 days. Two days after sertraline was discontinued, venlafaxine was started (37.5 mg twice daily for 12 days then increased to 75 mg twice daily). Concurrent medications included oxitropium and becloforte inhalers for asthma. Cognitive dysfunction progressed and was accompanied by postural hypotension (95/50 mmHg), myoclonic jerking, and difficulty walking. Abnormal laboratory tests included erythrocyte sedimentation rate (41 mm/hr), hyponatremia (123 mmol/L) and a plasma and urine osmolality of 269 mOsmol/kg and 852 mOsmol/kg, respectively. This profile suggested syndrome of inappropriate antidiuretic hormone secretion (SIADH). EEG performed at this time demonstrated slow wave activity without normal alpha rhythm. Although serum sodium levels normalized after five days of fluid restriction, symptoms continued during venlafaxine therapy (cumulative five weeks of therapy). Symptoms significantly improved over a six day period after venlafaxine was stopped. However, two weeks later, symptoms recurred within 48 hours after starting amitriptyline therapy (50 mg twice daily). Confusion reversed and myoclonic jerking improved over an eight day period after amitriptyline was discontinued. EEG performed at this time was improved.

The authors noted that this is the first report of relapsed serotonin syndrome with amitriptyline and that a two week washout period between the treatments suggested that the two episodes of serotonin effects were separate. Both agents are known to increase serotonergic activity.

Perry NK (Med for the Elderly, Poole Hosp NHS Trust, Longfleet Rd, Poole, Dorset BH15 2JB, UK) Venlafaxine induced serotonin syndrome with relapse following amitriptyline. Postgrad Med J 76:254–256 (Apr) 2000

ANTIPSYCHOTICS
ANTIPSYCHOTICS
In Utero Exposure: Neonatal Heart Block

A baby boy was delivered via Caesarean section during the 35th week of gestation due to fetal bradycardia and preterm labor. During pregnancy the mother took several antipsychotic medications for schizophrenia, including chlorpromazine, haloperidol and akineton (no dosages provided). She also had electroconvulsive therapy with the last session administered two days prior to delivery. Immediately after delivery the child was bradycardic (80 to 90 beats/min) with poor respirations, requiring intensive care admission. Physical examination was otherwise unremarkable. An electrocardiogram revealed a second-degree heart block and prolonged QTc interval (0.6 seconds). However, an echocardiogram demonstrated a structurally sound and normal heart. Within 24 hours the pulse rate increased from 50 to 60 beats/minute to 90 beats/minute without therapy, and to 120 to 130 beats/minute after 48 hours. At this time, QTc interval was within normal ranges.

The authors suggested that this neonatal transient heart block and prolonged QTc were related to maternal antipsychotic treatment or electroconvulsive therapy. A mechanism of action was not proposed. The authors also suggested that neonates born to pregnant women taking antipsychotics should be carefully monitored after delivery.

Ergenekon E et al (Yesilyurt Sokak No: 19/9, Cankaya 06690, Anakara, Turkey; e-mail:ergene@neuron.ato.org.tr) Transient heart block in a newborn due to maternal antipsychotic treatment during pregnancy. Eur J Pediatrics 159:137–138 (Jan/Feb) 2000

CHLORPROMAZINE
Corneal Deposits, Cataracts

A 50-year-old patient experienced gradual vision deterioration over a one-year period while taking chronic medications which included chlorpromazine (300 mg daily), trifluoperazine (10 mg daily), and trihexyphenidyl (4 mg daily). An ophthalmological examination revealed decreased visual acuity of 20/35 and 20/50 in the right and left eyes, respectively. Although a slit lamp examination exhibited refractile corneal deposits, intraocular pressures were normal in both eyes.

The authors concluded that chlorpromazine was responsible for corneal deposits and cataracts in this patient. A mechanism of action was not provided.

Leung ATS et al (Lam DSC, Dept Ophthalmology & Visual Sciences, Chinese Univ of Hong Kong, Prince of Wales Hosp, Shatin, New Territories, Hong Kong, China; e-mail:dennislam@cuhk.edu.hk) Chlorpromazine induced refractile corneal deposits and cataract. Arch Ophthalmol 117:1662–1663 (Dec) 1999 (letter)

CLOZAPINE
Stuttering

A 49-year-old psychiatric patient developed stuttering after her clozapine dosage was increased from 600 mg daily to 700 mg daily. EEG abnormalities were also noted but disappeared when the dose was decreased to 650 mg daily. However, stuttering symptoms recurred when the clozapine dose was increased again to treat a psychotic episode. At 750 mg daily, the patient experienced a generalized epileptic seizure requiring hospitalization and treatment with phenytoin. Once the clozapine dosage was reduced to 600 mg daily stuttering symptoms resolved and EEG changes normalized. Valproate (900 mg daily) was substituted for phenytoin. At a six-month follow-up the patient remained stabilized without seizures or symptoms.

The authors concluded that this patient experienced dose related clozapine induced stuttering as a result of epileptic brain activity. Based on this theory, they suggested that all patients who develop stuttering while on clozapine therapy should undergo EEG monitoring for brain epileptic activity.

Supprian T et al (Wurzburg, Germany) Clozapine induced stuttering: epileptic brain activity. Am J Psychiatry 156(10):1663–1664 (Oct) 1999

CLOZAPINE
Interstitial Nephritis (First Report*)

A 38-year-old woman was hospitalized for acute renal failure approximately 11 days after starting olanzapine therapy (125 mg twice daily). Other concurrent medications included lithium (750 mg daily) and venlafaxine (150 mg twice daily). Various mood stabilizers were also used over the previous year to stabilize the patient and included trifluperazine, fluphenazine and sertraline. Upon admission to the hospital symptoms included but were not limited to anorexia, lethargy, drowsiness, vomiting and a significant decrease in urination. Laboratory values were consistent with renal failure and included elevated urea (32.9 mmol/L), and creatinine (1.2 mmol/L). Trough lithium concentrations taken three weeks prior to admission were low but in therapeutic range (0.5 mmol/L). All drugs were stopped upon admission. Renal biopsy revealed interstitial infiltrates containing eosinophils consistent with drug induced renal problems. Hemodialysis was required four times during the first week of hospitalization with gradual increases in urine output by the end of the first week. Serum creatinine was within normal limits approximately two weeks after clozapine was stopped.

The authors noted that this was the first published report of clozapine induced acute interstitial nephritis, most likely due to an allergic response. They encouraged clinicians to monitor renal function in addition to potential bone marrow toxicity in patients receiving clozapine therapy.

Elias TJ et al (Dept Renal Med, Royal Adelaide Hosp, North Terrace, Adelaide 5000, Australia) Clozapine induced acute interstitial nephritis. Lancet 354:1180–1181 (Oct 2) 1999 (letter)

CLOZAPINE
Venous Thromboembolism

A review of adverse events reported to the Swedish Adverse Reactions Advisory Committee between April 1989 to March 2000 revealed six cases each of pulmonary embolism and venous thrombosis associated with clozapine therapy (mean dose: 277 mg daily). The mean age of the 12 patients was 38 yrs (range: 25 to 59 years) and the majority were men (77%). Symptoms occurred within the first three months in the majority of patients (67%) and resulted in death in five patients (42%). Only one patient (on concurrent oral contraceptives) had predisposing risk factors for venous thromboembolism.

The authors concluded that venous thromboembolism was associated with the use of clozapine in these patients and that potentially fatal events may occur within the first three months of use. They cautioned clinicians to discontinued clozapine when this reaction is suspected.

Hagg S et al (Div Clin Pharmacol, Norrland Univ Hosp, s-901 85 Umea, Sweden; email:staffan.hagg@pharm.umu.se) Association of venous thromboembolism and clozapine. Lancet 355:1155–1156 (Apr 1) 2000 (letter)

CLOZAPINE
Diabetes Mellitus

Two reports of patients who developed diabetes mellitus during clozapine therapy are described.

Patient 1: A 45-year-old patient with schizophrenia refractory to typical antipsychotics developed hyperglycemia (173 mg/dL) approximately 17 months after starting clozapine (900 mg daily). Initial management with diet restrictions were not successful and glyburide therapy was initiated approximately two years later (2.5 mg daily) and eventually titrated to 20 mg daily. Metformin (500 mg twice daily) was also added to his regimen. Hemoglobin A1c concentrations ranged from a low of 6.9 early in therapy to 9.2 after three years of clozapine therapy. Weight increase over this same period was 23 kg, resulting in 53% over ideal body weight. Other concurrent drugs after starting hypoglycemic therapy included magnesium hydroxide, ranitidine, prazosin, docusate, famotidine, albuterol, ipratropium (metered dose inhaler), ferrous sulfate, pseudoephedrine, amoxicillin, and dextromethorphan-guaifenesin syrup. No dosages were provided.

Patient 2: A 54-year-old patient with schizophrenia had repeated elevated glucose levels in the two years after starting clozapine therapy. Baseline serum glucose measurements (125 mg/dL) increased to as high as 193 mg/dL during five years of therapy, at which time glipizide was initiated (5 to 10 mg daily). Hemoglobin A1c concentrations ranged from a low of 5.4 early in therapy to 8.8 after seven years of clozapine therapy. Weight increase over this same period was 24.4 kg, resulting in 56.6% over ideal body weight. Other concurrent medications after clozapine was started included docusate, naproxen, diazepam, metoprolol, simvastatin, psyllium, nitroglycerin, levofloxacin, fludrocortisone, and lisinopril. The maintenance dose of clozapine was 800 mg daily.

The authors suggested that these patients developed diabetes mellitus as a result of clozapine induced weight gain. It was noted that both patients did not experience sudden changes in glycemic control after starting clozapine. However, both patients did gain excessive weight during clozapine therapy. The authors recommended that patients taking clozapine therapy should be closely monitored for impaired glucose tolerance and diabetes mellitus

Wehring H et al (Clin & Administrative Pharmacy Div, Coll Pharmacy, Univ Iowa, S-413 Pharmacy Bldg, Iowa City, IA 52242-1112) Diabetes mellitus associated with clozapine therapy. Pharmacotherapy 20(7).844–847 (Jul) 2000

CLOZAPINE, OLANZAPINE
Recurrent Priapism

A 43-year-old patient experienced two separate painful episodes of priapism during clozapine therapy for refractory psychosis (no dosage provided). Each episode lasted approximately 12 to 13 hours. After clozapine was withdrawn, priapism did not recur during substituted therapy with divalproex (1 gram daily) with olanzapine (25 mg daily) or thiothixene (5 mg daily). However, noncompliance with this regimen resulted in hospitalization for psychosis exacerbation. The morning after this therapy regimen was reinitiated the patient experienced another episode of painful priapism which resolved within eight to 10 hours. Olanzapine was discontinued and thiothixene dose was increased to 25 mg daily.

The authors noted that this was the third published report of olanzapine induced priapism, most likely due to the alpha adrenergic properties of both drugs. They cautioned clinicians to consider this possible risk when prescribing these agents in patients with a prior history of priapism.

Compton MT et al (Atlanta, GA) Recurrent priapism during treatment with clozapine and olanzapine. Am J Psychiatry 157(4):659 (Apr) 2000 (letter)

CLOZAPINE
Weight Gain, Lipid Abnormalities

In a five year prospective study, 82 patients on clozapine therapy for at least one year were monitored to determine the incidence of treatment emergent diabetes related to weight gain, lipid abnormalities, age, clozapine dosage and/or valproate use. During the study period, approximately half of the patients (52.4%) experienced at least one episode of elevated fasting blood glucose (>140 mg/dL) and 30% were diagnosed with adult onset type 2 diabetes mellitus. Approximately 67% of the patients experienced at least one episode of elevated fasting blood glucose equal to or above 126 mg/dL. Weight significantly increased over time among all 82 patients and was significantly correlated with change in total serum cholesterol and serum triglycerides. However, weight gain was not related to daily clozapine dosage or diabetes treatment. Weight gain was continuous until month 46 and then leveled off.

The authors concluded that this study demonstrated a high rate of weight gain and new onset diabetes mellitus in patients receiving clozapine therapy. Although an exact mechanism for these events is not known, proposed theories included clozapine suppression of insulin release, insulin resistance or impaired glucose utilization. The authors encouraged clinicians to monitor weight and blood pressures monthly.

Henderson DC et al (Freedom Trail Clinic, Harvard Med Sch, 25 Staniford St, Boston, MA 02114; e-mail:hend@med.mit.edu) Clozapine, diabetes mellitus, weight gain, and lipid abnormalities: a five year naturalistic study. Am J Psychiatry 157:975–981 (Jun) 2000

HALOPERIDOL
Dispensing Error, Overdose, Legal Action

A 38-year-old Tourette's patient claimed that his prescription for haloperidol was refilled with tablets that represented a tenfold increase over the correct dosage (5 mg tablets vs 0.5 mg tablets). After taking three tablets of the higher strength tablet the patient fainted and during transportation to the hospital jumped from the vehicle. The pharmacy noted liability after sample testing validated the error, but contended that the plaintiff was negligent in taking three tablets. The plaintiff claimed that the event led to worsening of Tourette's, suffering a post-traumatic stress disorder, development of nightmares and significant weight loss. The jury award for the plaintiff and wife was $383,300.

Davi vs Hook-Superx Inc, Revco Drug Center, CVS Pharmacy. Haldol prescription was ten times the proper dosage—man with Tourette's syndrome suffers overdose-post-traumatic stress disorder—New York court directs verdict for plaintiff on liability—jury

136 CNS

awards $383,300. Med Malpractice Verdicts, Settlements & Experts 16(8):48–49 (Aug) 2000

HALOPERIDOL AND IMIPENEM
Hypotension with Intravenous Administration

Three cases of hypotension are described with concurrent haloperidol and imipenem regimens.

Patient 1: A 75-year-old woman developed hypotension (65/34 mmHg) within 15 minutes after intravenous haloperidol was administered (0.5 mg). At 30 minutes after administration blood pressure was 103/30 mmHg and heart rate was 120 bpm. Concurrent medications included intravenous imipenem (500 mg every six hours), albuterol (two puffs four times daily), ipratropium bromide, subcutaneous heparin (5000 units twice daily), methylprednisolone (60 mg daily), erythromycin (500 mg every six hours) and famotidine (20 mg twice daily).

Patient 2: A 56-year-old inpatient developed hypotension (91/49 mmHg) approximately 15 minutes after haloperidol was administered intravenously (2.5 mg). At 30 minutes, blood pressure was 100/57 mmHg. Concurrent medications included intravenous meperidine (25–50 mg every four hours as needed) and intravenous fluids.

Patient 3: A 43-year-old inpatient with developed hypotension (91/50 mmHg) with a heart rate of 92 bpm after intravenous administration of haloperidol which increased to 94/55 mmHg at 30 minutes and 107/66 mmHg at 60 minutes post infusion. Concurrent medications included intravenous erythromycin (500 mg every six hours), intravenous imipenem (500 mg daily), albuterol, TPN, intravenous famotidine (20 mg twice daily) and midazolam (as needed).

The authors noted that all three patients had stabilized blood pressures while on imipenem therapy prior to intravenous haloperidol administration. Hypotension in these patients was transient and reversed within an hour. Only one patient required treatment with dopamine (patient 1). The authors suggested that a drug interaction may have increased free serum concentration of haloperidol causing a hypotensive effect.

Franco-Bronson K & Gajwani P (Cleveland Clin Foundation, Dept Psychiatry & Psychology, Cleveland OH 44195) Hypotension associated with intravenous haloperidol and imipenem. J Clin Psychopharmacol 19(5):480–481 (Oct) 1999 (letter)

LITHIUM
Asthma Precipitation Upon Drug Discontinuation
(First Report*)

A 37-year-old man developed nocturnal coughing and exertional wheezing approximately six weeks after long term lithium was discontinued

(1400 mg daily for 14 years). Airway responsiveness increased accompanied by significant decreases in FEV-1 values (112 to 66) after the drug was stopped. Concurrent medication included sulpiride (600 mg daily). Symptoms improved with inhaled budesonide and terbutaline therapy. When inhaled therapy was stopped several months later, asthma symptoms recurred.

The authors noted that this was the first case report of asthma occurring post-lithium withdrawal. Although an exact mechanism of action was not provided, it was noted that asthma symptoms have improved while on lithium therapy.

Convery RP et al (Whiston Hosp, Prescot, Merseyside L35 5DR, UK) Asthma precipitated by cessation of lithium treatment. Postgrad Med J 75:637–638 (Oct) 1999

OLANZAPINE
Excessive Weight Gain

A 17-year-old adolescent gained approximately 20 pounds over a six-month period while taking olanzapine (5 mg daily) for schizophrenia. An additional 16.5 pounds were gained during a seven week period at a higher dosage level (10 mg daily). Diet and activity level were unaltered during these periods. After a total of 14 months of olanzapine therapy, a total weight gain of 85 pounds had occurred with a 58% increase in body mass index (32.9 mg/kg 2). Initial substitution with quetiapine (400 mg dally) was unsuccessful in controlling schizophrenia symptoms, but symptoms responded to risperidone therapy (2 mg daily). At 19.5 years of age, the patient had lost 15 pounds once olanzapine was stopped.

The authors concluded that although olanzapine associated weight gain has been reported, this was the first case report of extreme weight gain in an adolescent. They proposed that H1 and 5-hydroxytryptamine 2-receptor antagonism might be responsible for weight gain associated with psychotropic agents.

Bryden KE & Kopala LC (Halifax, Nova Scotia, Canada) Body mass index increase of 58% associated with olanzapine. Am J Psychiatry 156 (11):1835–1836 (Nov) 1999 (letter)

RISPERIDONE
Meige's Syndrome

A 43-year-old psychiatric patient developed episodic blepharospasms after recently being switched from thioridazine therapy (50 mg daily) which he had been taking for approximately six years, to risperidone (6 mg daily). Although the patient had taken various neuroleptics on a chronic basis, he was not taking other medications at the time the problem developed. Unfortunately, the blepharospasms occurred with and without triggers, resulting in significant change in life style (e.g., discontinuing driving).

The authors concluded that this patient's blepharospasms (Meige's Syndrome) were caused by risperidone. Although an exact mechanism of action was not provided, the authors noted that other neuroleptics have been associated with this syndrome and that drug withdrawal usually results in reversal.

Ananth J et al. Meige's syndrome associated with risperidone therapy. Am J Psychiatry 157:149 (Jan) 2000 (letter)

RISPERIDONE
Tardive Dyskinesia

A 16-year-old patient with paranoid schizophrenia developed involuntary buccolingual masticatory movements, and non-repetitive movements of the arms and fingers after several months of risperidone therapy (titrated up to 4 mg daily). Prior to and during risperidone therapy she had also received small dosages of other typical antipsychotics. Involuntary movements worsened over the next eight months after risperidone dosage was increased (6 mg daily). The addition of trifluoperazine (10 mg daily for six months) was unsuccessful and discontinued. Unresponsive to two doses of flupenthixol depot (20 mg) with worsening of psychotic symptoms resulted in hospitalization. Risperidone was restarted at 2 mg daily and titration up to 6 mg resulted in improved tardive dyskinesia. The patient remained disease and symptom free during a 12-month follow-up.

The authors proposed that tardive dyskinesia in this patient was related to risperidone therapy based on the temporal relationship between drug administration and symptoms. They also noted that the reversal of symptoms when risperidone was reintroduced at lower dosages has also been reported with other typical antipsychotics.

Kumar S & Malone DM (Lakeland Health Ltd, Private bag 3023, Rotorua, New Zealand; email:shailesh.kumar@clear.net.nz) Risperidone implicated in the onset of tardive dyskinesia in a young woman. Postgrad Med J 76:316–317 (May) 2000

RISPERIDONE
Reduced Incidence of Tardive Dyskinesia

In a one year open label study, 330 patients with dementia of various etiologies (mean age: 82.5 yrs) were monitored for the incidence of tardive dyskinesia while receiving various doses of risperidone (0.5 mg to 2 mg daily). The majority of patients were women (69.1%) with dementia related to Alzheimer's disease (76%). The mean dose of risperidone was 0.96 mg daily for a median of 273 days. Of the 255 patients without dyskinesia at baseline, 2.6% developed dyskinesia. The emergence of persistent tardive dyskinesia may have been dose related as dyskinesia occurred in four patients who received greater than 1.5 mg daily and in 2 patients who received doses ranging from 0.75 mg to 1.5 mg daily. However, there were no cases observed in patients receiving less than 0.75 mg daily. In addition, of the 59 patients with dyskinesia at baseline, approximately half (49.2%) demonstrated improvement in all five dyskinesia factors including dyskinetic movements, hyperkinesia, buccolingual mastication, choreoathetosis in limbs, and dyskinesia.

The authors concluded that the observed incidence of persistent tardive dyskinesia with risperidone was lower than expected or reported in elderly patients who have been treated with conventional neuroleptics.

Jeste DV et al (Dr. Martinez, Janssen Pharmaceutica and Research Foundation, 1125 Trenton—Harbourton Rd, Titusville, NJ 08560; e-mail:rmartin@janus. jnj.com) Low incidence of persistent tardive dyskinesia in elderly patients with dementia treated with risperidone. Am J Psychiatry 157:1150–1155 (Jul) 2000

THIORIDAZINE
QT Prolongation, FDA Advisory

On July 7, 2000, the manufacturer (Novartis Pharmaceuticals Corporation) of thioridazine notified health professionals regarding new labeling changes in the product insert. Specifically, a boxed warning has been added regarding the potential for dose related QTc prolongation, torsades de pointes and sudden death. The drug is now limited for use only for schizophrenic patients who fail to show an acceptable response to adequate courses of treatment with other antipsychotic drugs, either because of insufficient effectiveness or the inability to achieve an effective dose due to intolerable adverse effects. Thioridazine is also now contraindicated with fluvoxamine, propranolol, pindolol, other cytochrome P450-2D6 inhibitors (e.g., fluoxetine and paroxetine), and drugs known to prolong the QTc interval. A baseline ECG and serum potassium should be performed prior to the initiation of and periodically during thioridazine therapy. Therapy should not be started if the QTc interval is longer than 450 msec and should be discontinued if the QTc interval is greater than 500 msec. These changes to the product labeling are based primarily on the FDA's review of three published studies.

New product labeling for thioridazine. (Jul) 2000. http://www.fda.gov/med-watch/ safety/ 2000/mellar.htm

SEDATIVE/HYPNOTICS
DIAZEPAM
Propylene Glycol Toxicity

A 46-year-old inpatient developed propylene glycol toxicity after receiving approximately 3000 mg of diazepam over 24 hours for alcohol withdrawal symptoms. Symptoms after diazepam administration included tachypnea and progressive hypotension. Arterial gas studies revealed a pH of 7.16, partial pressure carbon dioxide of 22 mmHg, and partial pressure oxygen of 90 mmHg. Bicarbonate levels decreased (7 mmol/L), and creatinine increased (2.2 mg/dL). Treatment included two vasopressor agents (nonspecified) and emergency dialysis. After only one dialysis session, the acid-base status returned to normal and recovery was uneventful. The propylene glycol level was 1300 mg/dL.

The authors concluded that acidosis developed in this patient as a result of high dose diazepam administration, resulting in excessive propylene glycol administration, which was metabolized to lactic acid.

Wilson KC et al (Boston Univ Sch Med, Boston, MA 02118–2394) Propylene glycol toxicity in a patient receiving intravenous diazepam. N Engl J Med 343(11):815–816 (Sep 14) 2000 (letter)

MIDAZOLAM
Paradoxical Reactions

The following case reports describe the unusual presentation of paradoxical reactions to midazolam when administered as a premedicant for gastrointestinal endoscopies in three adults. In all patients the reactions reversed with the administration of flumazenil.

Patient 1: A 62-year-old man developed a paradoxical reaction after receiving meperidine (12.5 mg) and midazolam (5 mg titrated slowly) as premedicants for gastrointestinal endoscopy. Despite adequate sedation, intubation was not possible because of patient resistance, head shaking and arm swinging. The administration of intravenous droperidol (5 mg) was unsuccessful in reducing this behavior. However, after the administration of intravenous flumazenil (0.5 mg) the patient remained sedated without disturbed behavior and intubation was successful. An uneventful endoscopy was performed without changes in blood pressure or oxygen saturation. The patient had no recollection of the procedure upon recovery.

Patient 2: A 58-year-old woman developed a paradoxical reaction after receiving meperidine (12.5 mg), droperidol (5 mg), and midazolam (7.5 mg titrated slowly) as premedicants for gastrointestinal endoscopy. Despite adequate sedation, the patient remained restless and agitated making intubation difficult. The administration of intravenous flumazenil (0.5 mg) resulted in rapid calming of the patient and allowed successful intubation. An uneventful endoscopy was performed without changes in blood pressure or oxygen saturation. The patient had no recollection of the procedure upon recovery.

Patient 3: A 26-year-old man developed a paradoxical reaction after receiving intravenous meperidine (25 mg), droperidol (5 mg), and midazolam (10 mg titrated slowly) as premedicants for gastrointestinal endoscopy.

Despite adequate sedation, the patient continually spit through the mouthpiece with repeated shaking of arms and legs. The administration of intravenous flumazenil (0.5 mg) resulted in rapid calming of the patient and allowed successful intubation. An uneventful endoscopy was performed without changes in blood pressure or oxygen saturation. The patient had no recollection of the procedure upon recovery.

The authors suggested that paradoxical reactions to benzodiazepines used for conscious sedation are not commonly reported. They also noted that only the aggressive behavior reversed in these cases while adequate sedation was maintained.

Fulton SA & Mulen KD (Dept Intern Med, Div Gastroenterol, Case Western Reserve Univ, Metrohealth Med Center, Cleveland, OH) Completion of upper endoscopic procedures despite paradoxical reaction to midazolam: a role for flumazenil? Am J Gastroenterol 95(3):809–811 (Mar) 2000

MIDAZOLAM, CHLORAL HYDRATE
Prolonged Recovery and Delayed Side Effects in Children

In an open study, 376 children (mean age: 3.8 yrs) who received sedation for outpatient diagnostic imaging procedures (either MRI or CT) were followed for prolonged sedation and delayed side effects. The most frequently used sedatives were chloral hydrate (80%) or midazolam (11%) alone, or in combination (9%). Children receiving chloral hydrate alone were significantly younger than those receiving midazolam alone or in combination (mean age: 2.9 vs 4.5 yrs). Inadequate sedation occurred more often in older children (mean age 4.8 vs 2.7 yrs) and most commonly with combined therapy (32%) when compared to sole therapy with midazolam (25%) or chloral hydrate (8%). Failed sedation was also more frequent in the combined sedative group (21%) when compared to midazolam (13%) or chloral hydrate alone (5%).

Approximately 51% of the children experienced prolonged sedation measured by sleeping during the ride home and 31% continued to sleep for at least six hours post-discharge. The most frequently cited adverse event during the hospital stay was gastrointestinal (2%) or agitation (2%). The incidences of post-discharge events were more frequent and included motor imbalance (31%), gastrointestinal (23%), agitation (19%), and restlessness (14%). Motor imbalance was significantly higher in the combined group (50%) than in either the midazolam or chloral hydrate alone groups (18% vs 31%, respectively). Agitation or aggression was also highest in the combined group (38% vs 18% vs 8%, respectively) and in 36% of the cases persisted for greater than six hours. Other less commonly cited symptoms included nausea/vomiting (13%), and diarrhea (11%). Less than half of the sedated children returned to baseline activity and behavior within eight hours after the procedure, 89% within 24 hours, and less than or equal to five percent within 48 hours. Infants (those less than 12 months) were more prone to delayed recovery when compared to older children.

The authors concluded that children may experience prolonged recovery and delayed side effects after sedation with chloral hydrate and/or midazolam for a diagnostic procedure. Younger patients were associated with a higher incidence of side effects.

Malviya S et al (Dept Anesthesiology, F3900/Box 0211, 1500 E Medical Center Drive, Ann Arbor, MI 48109-0211; e-mail:smalviya@umich.ed) Prolonged recovery and delayed side effects of sedation for diagnostic imaging studies in children. Pediatrics 105(3):42–46.

ZOLPIDEM
CNS Effects

Three case reports described central nervous system reactions in patients taking zolpidem. Side effects included disturbing nightmares, confusion, unsteady gait, and vomiting.

Patient 1: A 20-year-old male patient was hospitalized with traumatic injuries suffered in a motor vehicle accident. Three nights after starting zolpidem (5 mg initially, increased to 10 mg nightly) for insomnia he experienced anxiety provoking nightmares. The nightmares resolved after the zolpidem was discontinued.

Patient 2: A 24-year-old female inpatient with orthopedic injuries awoke disoriented and confused approximately three hours after taking a zolpidem dose for insomnia (10 mg). Concurrent medications included paroxetine and acetaminophen with codeine. Mental status varied during the following six hours but returned to baseline by morning. Paroxetine and zolpidem were discontinued without further event. Paroxetine was restarted without further incident.

Patient 3: A 26-year-old female patient developed nausea, vomiting, shaking and unsteady gait within 20 minutes after taking the first dose of zolpidem (10 mg) on an empty stomach with water. There were no concurrent medications. Additional symptoms included visual hallucinations, erratic speech patterns and difficulty understanding speech of others. The symptoms were transient in nature and lasted only 30 minutes, resolving when the patient fell asleep.

The authors noted that hallucinations, delirium or nightmares may be uncommon reactions to zolpidem. They also suggested that zolpidem toxicity may be influenced by the dose, patient's gender, protein binding and cytochrome P450 isoenzyme inhibition. Higher doses, particularly in women have been associated with increased plasma levels (by 40%) and may be associated with a higher incidence of side effects. The authors also suggested that zolpidem high protein binding affinity may be displaced if used with another drug that is highly protein bound. In addition, zolpidem is extensively metabolized by cytochrome P450 3A4 isoenzyme system and inhibition of this pathway by other drugs may increase the likelihood of toxicity. The authors recommended that clinicians consider these variables when prescribing zolpidem to minimize side effects.

Toner CL et al (Catalano G, Univ South Florida Psychiatry Center, 3515 E Fletcher Ave, Tampa, FL 33613) Central nervous system side effects associated with zolpidem treatment. Clin Neuropharmacol 23:54–58 (Feb) 2000

MISCELLANEOUS
CYCLOBENZAPRINE
Hallucinations

A 76-year-old patient developed hallucinations several weeks after starting cyclobenzaprine (10 mg four times daily) for muscle spasms associated with rheumatoid arthritis. Other chronic medications included ibuprofen, hydrocodone with acetaminophen, phenylpropanolamine, omeprazole, verapamil, albuterol, cyanocobalamin, ascorbic acid, cod liver oil, ferrous sulfate, and extended release potassium chloride (no dosages provided). Within 24 to 48 hours after cyclobenzaprine was discontinued, mental status improved.

The authors concluded that this elderly patient developed symptoms suggestive of central nervous stimulation as a result of cyclobenzaprine therapy. They suggested that the elderly may be more susceptible to adverse events based on organ function changes and an increased risk of drug interactions as a result of polypharmacy.

Douglass MA & Levine D (Detroit, MI) Hallucinations in an elderly patient taking recommended doses of cyclobenzaprine. Arch Intern Med 160:1373 (May 8) 2000 (letter)

NALTREXONE
Opioid Withdrawal Syndrome

A 35-year-old woman developed an unsteady gait, dizziness and visual hallucinations approximately one hour after receiving oral naltrexone (12.5 mg) for cholestatic pruritus. Although severe in nature, the reaction lasted only about 2.5 hours. A similar but shorter reaction (lasting 1.25 hours) occurred upon rechallenge with a lower dose of the drug (2 mg) four weeks later. In addition, generalized pruritus also developed. Approximately seven months later, she was hospitalized for a naloxone infusion (0.002 mcg/kg/min) which was increased to 0.2 mcg/kg/min over the next five days. Generalized paresthesia and mild pruritus developed. Oral naltrexone was substituted (12.5 mg twice dally) without reaction and continued for the next 12 months without symptoms.

The authors noted that this patient had a withdrawal type reaction to initial therapy with naltrexone for cholestatic pruritus. They also suggested that this reaction might be minimized by starting with a naloxone infusion titrated to therapeutic range and then substituting naltrexone therapy.

Jones EA & Dekker LRC (Depts GI & Liver Diseases, Academic Med Center, 1105 AZ Amsterdam-ZO,The Netherlands; e-mail: E.A.Jones@amc.uva.nl) Florid opioid withdrawal like reaction precipitated by naltrexone in a patient with chronic cholestasis. Gastroenterology 118: 431–432 (Feb) 2000

EENT

EENT

EENT

EENT

EENT

EENT

Drug	Interacting Drug	ADR	Page Number
Beta-blockers (ocular)		Ocular side effects	147
Brimonidine		Psychosis*	148
Dextromethorphan	Pseudoephedrine	Psychosis	148
Dextromethorphan		Psychosis	149
Latanoprost		Intraocular pressure (increased)	150
Latanoprost		Eyelash formation	150
Pseudoephedrine		Ischemic colitis	151
Pseudoephedrine	Dextromethorphan	Psychosis	148
Timolol		Respiratory arrest (+)	151
Unoprostone		Intraocular pressure (increased)	150
* = first report (+) = legal action			

EENT

BETA-BLOCKERS (Ocular)
Incidence of Ocular Side Effects

A survey of practicing ophthalmologists in the Netherlands over a three month period assessed the incidence of ocular side effects associated with the use of ocular beta-blockers. A total of 328 ophthalmologists participated, representing 70% of the practitioners in the Netherlands. During the study, 34 patients (mean age: 71.3 yrs) reported ocular side effects during beta-blocker use for a median duration of 14 months (range: 1 to 144 months). Five patients were also on concurrent ocular glaucoma agents. Clinical improvement occurred in all followed patients (28) after discontinuation of the drug or change in drug therapy. The most frequently reported side effects involved the eyelids (44%) as periorbital dermatitis or blepharitis, the conjunctiva (21%), or both (23%). Four patients (12%) experienced corneal involvement as punctate keratitis. However, no cases of uveitis were observed. The ocular medications most commonly cited included timolol (12 cases), levobunolol (5), betaxolol (4), metipranolol (4), carteolol (3), and bufenolol (1). The calculated incidence of ocular side effects associated with topical beta-blockers was 1.51 cases per 1000 patient years. Calculated incidence rates (cases/1000 patient years) for different beta-blockers ranged from 0.82 for betaxolol to 5.24 for bufenolol.

The authors concluded that ocular beta-blocker therapy is not associated with significant ocular adverse effects in the clinical setting. They suggested that this safety profile should be considered when comparing ocular beta-blockers to other topical glaucoma agents.

Van Beek LM et al. (Leiden Univ Med Center, Dept Ophthalmol, PO Box 9600, 2300 RN Leiden, Netherlands; e-mail:lmvanbeek@lumc.nl) Incidence of ocular side effects of topical beta-blockers in Netherlands. Br J Ophthalmol 84:856–859 (Aug) 2000

BRIMONIDINE
Psychosis (First Report*)

A 68-year-old patient without prior psychiatric history developed significant behavioral changes approximately three months after starting ocular brimonidine therapy for mild open angle glaucoma. No other medications were mentioned. Symptoms included fatigue, depression, and anxiety, progressing to delusions and severe confusion. Upon physical examination visual acuity was 20/20 and intraocular pressures were 16 mmHg and 14 mmHg in the right and left eyes, respectively. Latanoprost (0.005%) ophthalmic solution was substituted for brimonidine. However, before the actual change in therapy was made, the patient was hospitalized for psychosis after brandishing a gun. Within 48 hours after brimonidine was discontinued the patient's behavior returned to baseline and delusions reversed.

The author noted that this is the first case report of brimonidine induced psychosis. No mechanism of action was proposed but the author suggested that patients should be counseled regarding possible drug induced behavioral changes.

Kim DD (Green Bay, WI) A case of suspected alphagan induced psychosis. Arch Ophthalmol 118;1132–1133 (Aug) 2000 (letter)

DEXTROMETHORPHAN AND PSEUDOEPHEDRINE
Psychosis

Three reports of severe acute psychosis are described in young patients who combined over the counter medications containing ephedrine/ pseudoephedrine and dextromethorphan.

Patient 1: A 15-year-old girl was admitted to the emergency room with a 48 hour history of acute psychosis, including confusion with auditory and visual hallucinations. Although she was taking no prescribed therapy, she had a history of prior drug and alcohol abuse. A urine drug screen was positive for ephedrine/ pseudoephedrine and the patient later vomited three tablets. Although laboratory values, lumbar puncture and CT head scans were within normal ranges, the patient remained agitated and depressed with visual hallucinations. Symptoms gradually resolved over a two-day period with treatment including risperidone (2 mg daily) and clonazepam (1.5 mg daily).

Patient 2: A 13-year-old girl developed acute behavioral changes over a three day period while taking a nonprescription product containing dextromethorphan (15 mg), pseudoephedrine (60 mg) and carbinoxamine (4 mg) once to twice daily for flu symptoms. Although CT head scan, EEG and brain MRI were within normal ranges, the patient remained agitated, paranoid, extremely irritable, and continued to experience auditory hallucinations. Symptoms improved with risperidone treatment (2 mg daily) and the patient was transferred to a psychiatry service. Some symptoms remained and olanzapine was substituted for risperidone (7.5 mg daily). The patient eventually left the hospital against medical advice.

Patient 3: A 10-year-old girl with asthma but without a prior history of psychiatric illness developed acute mental status changes requiring hospitalization. Medications included pseudoephedrine (15 mg as needed), prednisone (120 mg daily tapered to 5 mg daily) azithromycin (no dosage provided) and nebulized albuterol. Symptoms included paranoia, confusion, irritability and hallucinations (auditory and visual). Scans and EEGs were within normal ranges, but symptoms remained for an additional five days after discontinuation of all medications. Some symptoms remained after discharge despite risperidone therapy (0.5 mg daily). However, irritability and thought process improved after a steroid inhaler was stopped.

The authors noted that each girl took a different nonprescription cold product containing pseudoephedrine/ephedrine with dextromethorphan and in some cases these products were combined with other medications. In addition, steroids may have contributed to the symptoms in patient 3. However, the authors proposed that the use of dextromethorphan/pseudoephedrine combination precipitated psychotic symptoms, requiring hospitalization and thorough medical evaluations. They also recommended that this combination be used with caution in children and adolescents.

Solute CA et al (Div Child & Adolescent Psychiatry, Children's Hosp Med Center, Cincinnati, Dept Psychiatry, Biol Psychiatry Program, Univ Cincinnati) Psychosis associated with pseudoephedrine and dextromethorphan. J Am Acad Chil Adolesc Psychiatry 38:1471–1472 (Dec) 1999 (letter)

DEXTROMETHORPHAN
Psychosis

An 18-year-old student was hospitalized for visual hallucinations and a depersonalization reaction after several days of ingesting one to two bottles of cough syrup, which contained dextromethorphan (711 mg/bottle). Although the student had a past history of attention deficit disorder and social phobia, he was taking no other medications at the time of admission. However, he admitted to intermittent marijuana use. Additional symptoms included delusions, paranoia, and disassociation, which all resolved within four days of admission without neuroleptic treatment. During the next two months he was rehospitalized with similar psychotic symptoms after ingesting large amounts of cough syrup. During these admissions, symptoms resolved without treatment.

The authors concluded that abuse of dextromethorphan was responsible for inducing psychotic symptoms in this patient. They noted that previous similar reports suggested symptoms were related to sympathomimetic ingredients. They cautioned clinicians to be aware of this potential abuse pattern with subsequent complications.

Price LH & Lebel J (Providence, RI) Dextromethorphan induced psychosis. Am J Psychiatry 157(2):304 (Feb) 2000 (letter)

LATANOPROST
Eyelash Formation

A 53-year-old patient with long term alopecia (loss of eyelashes and diffuse scalp hair for five years) experienced eyelash regrowth within three weeks after latanoprost for glaucoma. Latanoprost was chosen for possible hypertrichosis effects. Two months after starting latanoprost, full growth of eyelashes was documented.

The authors concluded that latanoprost was responsible for eyelash regrowth in this patient, possibly related to prostaglandin F2a stimulation in hair cells. The authors suggested that clinicians should be aware of this possible effect. Mansberger SL & Cioffi GA. (Devers Eye Instit/Discoveries in Sight, 1040 NW 22nd

Ave, Suite 200, Portland, OR 97210) Eyelash formation secondary to latanoprost treatment in a patient with alopecia. Arch Ophthalmol 118:718–719 (May) 2000 (letter)

LATANOPROST, UNOPROSTONE
Increased Intraocular Pressure (First Reports*)

A 29-year-old woman with retinitis pigmentosa developed increased intraocular pressures (IOPs: 30 to 56 mmHg) and corneal edema within 24 hours after unoprostone administration (two drops once). IOPs returned to 15 mmHg after unoprostone therapy was stopped and ranged between one and 35 mmHg during a follow-up period of several weeks. Five months later, similar IOP increases (55 mmHg) and corneal edema occurred after latanoprost administration. IOPs returned to baseline levels after latanoprost was withdrawn. Although repeated diode laser cyclophotocoagulation treatments initially reduced IOPs (range: 10 to 20 mmHg), they decreased to 0 mmHg five months after the last laser treatment. IOPs increased to 55 mmHg within 36 hours after two drops of unoprostone was applied.

The authors noted that these were the first reports of IOP increases associated with unoprostone and latanoprost administration. They suggested that impaired trabecular outflow in this patient may have contributed to this event.

Ness T & Funk J (Univ Augenklinik Freiburg, Killianstr. 5, D-79106 Freiburg, Germany) Increase of intraocular pressure after topical administration of prostaglandin analogs. Arch Ophthalmol 117:1646–1647 (Dec) 1999 (letter)

PSEUDOEPHEDRINE
Ischemic Colitis

A 33-year-old man developed abdominal cramping, diarrhea and hematochezia approximately 3 days after starting pseudoephedrine extended release tablets (120 mg twice daily) for nasal decongestion. Concurrent medications included long term albuterol and corticosteroid inhalers for chronic asthma (no dosages provided). The pseudoephedrine was stopped after five days of therapy. Colonoscopy revealed patchy erythema and mucosal edema in the descending colon. Colonic biopsy also revealed necrosis, edema and hemorrhage indicative of ischemic colitis. Infectious, immunologic and thromboembolic etiologies were ruled out via laboratory testing. Symptoms resolved after discontinuation of pseudoephedrine and did not recur within a 10 month follow—up period.

The authors concluded that pseudoephedrine may be a risk factor for ischemic colitis and suggested that case control studies were needed to assess the potential causal relationship.

Lichtenstein GR & Yee NS (Hosp Univ Penn, Philadelphia, PA 19104-4283) Ischemic colitis associated with decongestant use. Ann Intern Med 132(8):682

TIMOLOL (Ocular)
Respiratory Arrest, Irreversible Brain Damage, Legal Action

An 81-year-old patient with glaucoma and asthma suffered a respiratory arrest after receiving ophthalmic timolol in the physician's office. Despite resuscitation efforts, the patient experienced irreversible brain damage, requiring nursing home care until her death four years later. A settlement of $900,000 was reached.

Anon 81 year old vs Anon Ophthalmologist. Failure to realize timolol was contraindicated for patients with respiratory problems—irreversible brain damage, coma and confinement to nursing home—Massachusetts settlement for $900,000. Med Malpractice Verdicts & Settlements & Experts 16(2):39 (Feb) 2000

GASTROINTESTINAL AGENTS
GASTROINTESTINAL AGENTS
GASTROINTESTINAL AGENTS
GASTROINTESTINAL AGENTS
GASTROINTESTINAL AGENTS
GASTROINTESTINAL AGENTS

Drug	Interacting Drug	ADR	Page Number
Alosetron		Ischemic colitis, constipation	155
Calcium carbonate		Milk-alkali syndrome	155
Calcium carbonate	Levothyroxine	Levothyroxine absorption reduced	156
Cisapride		Cardiac toxicity	
Cisapride		Market withdrawal due to ADRs	158
Cisapride	Grapefruit juice	Cisapride concentrations increased	157
Infliximab		Increased susceptibility to Listeriosis*	158
Misoprostol		Contraindication in pregnancy	159
Omeprazole		Interstitial nephritis	160
Omeprazole	Clarithromycin	Omeprazole concentrations increased	159
Ondansetron		Myocardial infarction	160
Phosphate enema		Hypocalcemia (infant)	161
Prochlorperazine		Akathisia	162
Proton pump inhibitors		Anaphylactic reactions	162
Psyllium		Bronchiolitis	163
Ranitidine		Toxic epidermal necrolysis	163
Sulfasalazine		Hemolyticanemia	164
* = first report			

Gastrointestinal Agents

ALOSETRON
FDA Advisory: Ischemic Colitis, Constipation

On August 24, 2000 Glaxo Wellcome and the FDA notified health professionals regarding new safety information for alosetron, a serotonin 5-HT3 antagonist approved in the United States for irritable bowel syndrome in women. New information refers to postmarketing reports of constipation and ischemic colitis. In some cases constipation has progressed to more serious events including obstruction, perforation, impaction, toxic megacolon, and secondary ischemia. Intestinal surgery (including colectomy) was warranted in some patients. The product information insert has been changed to emphasize this new information. Alosetron therapy should not be initiated in patients with constipation and is contraindicated in patients with a history of severe or chronic constipation, in patients who have had a history of complications caused by constipation, and in patients with a history of intestinal obstruction, stricture, toxic megacolon, gastrointestinal perforation and/or adhesions. Additional contraindications also include active diverticulitis, a history of ischemic colitis, or current or past Crohn's disease or ulcerative colitis. A new medication guide for patients has also been published.

Safety related revisions to labeling for Lotronex (alosetron hydrochloride) tablets. Important new dispensing information: Issuance of a patient medication guide. (Aug 23) 2000. http://www.fda.gov/medwatch/safety/2000/lotron.htm

CALCIUM CARBONATE
Milk Alkali Syndrome

A 44-year-old patient was hospitalized with symptoms of abdominal pain and vomiting. No medications were mentioned during a medication history at admission. Additional symptoms included drowsiness, dehydration, tachycardia (110 beats per minute) and hypertension (160/110 mmHg). Abnormal laboratory values included elevated BUN (11.4 mmol/L), alkaline phosphatase (163 IU/L), creatinine (216 umol/L), amylase (3500 U/L), and corrected calcium (4.0 mmol/L). The patient was diagnosed with pancreatitis secondary to milk alkali syndrome. Although the patient initially denied medication use, a repeat medication history revealed the chronic use of nonprescription calcium-containing antacids for the last two to three years for osteoporosis prevention. Each antacid tablet contained 680 mg calcium carbonate. Approximate weekly intake averaged 70 tablets a week or 4.5 grams of calcium carbonate daily. Recovery was uneventful after therapy with lansoprazole (20 mg daily) was initiated. Post-discharge follow-up revealed electrolyte values that had returned to baseline levels.

George S & Clark JDA (Addenbrookes Hosp NHS Trust, Cambridge, UK; e-mail: John.Clark@wsh—tr.anglox.nhs.uk) Milk alkali syndrome—an unusual syndrome causing an unusual complication. Postgrad Med J 76:422–423 (Jul) 2000

CALCIUM CARBONATE AND LEVOTHYROXINE
Interaction: T4 Absorption Reduced

In a prospective one-year cohort study, 20 adult patients with hypothyroidism stabilized on chronic levothyroxine therapy, ingested calcium carbonate (1200 mg daily of elemental calcium) for three months. At the end of three months, free T4 serum concentrations and total T4 were significantly decreased when compared to baseline (1.34 vs 1.22 ng/dL and 9.21 vs 8.55 mcg/dL). In contrast, mean thyroid stimulating hormone concentrations were significantly increased (1.6 vs 2.71 mIU/L). Mean T3 serum concentrations, however, were unchanged during concurrent administration of the two products (141.50 vs 142.10 ng/dL). All values returned to near baseline levels at two months after calcium carbonate administration was discontinued.

The authors concluded that calcium carbonate has a clinically moderate but significant impact on thyroid function. They suggested that the decrease in levothyroxine's bioavailability is mediated by levothyroxine adsorption to calcium carbonate in an acidic environment. Clinicians are advised to monitor any changes in thyroid function tests in patients who are taking both calcium carbonate and levothyroxine. Separating administration times was advised.

Singh N et al. (Div Endocrinol & Metabolism, Endocrinology 111D, VA Greater Los Angeles Healthcare System, 11301 Wilshire Blvd, Los Angeles, CA 90073; e-mail: nsingh@ucla.edu) Effect of calcium carbonate on the absorption of levothyroxine.

CISAPRIDE AND GRAPEFRUIT JUICE
Interaction: Increased Cisapride Concentrations

In a randomized crossover study, 10 healthy male volunteers (age range: 21-31 years) ingested either water or double strength grapefruit juice (200 mL three times daily) for three days. On day three, a single dose of cisapride (10 mg) was administered in the morning. An additional 200-mL of fluid was ingested 0.5 and 1.5 hours after cisapride administration. A washout period of two weeks separated the trials. When taken with grapefruit juice, several cisapride kinetic parameters were increased including, maximum concentrations (78.3 vs 43.2 ng/mL), time to maximum concentration (2.5 vs 1.5 hrs), half-life (8.4 vs 6.8 hrs) and area under the curve (889 vs 365 ng/mL/hr). Monitoring of QTc intervals post cisapride dosing revealed that in both groups, the QTc interval at five hours was significantly prolonged when compared to baseline. However, grapefruit juice did not significantly increase QTc intervals when compared to the control group at any time.

The authors concluded that grapefruit juice significantly increased cisapride plasma concentrations most likely via selective inhibition of CYP3A4 metabolism. The amount and brand of grapefruit juice may effect the degree of the grapefruit/drug interaction.

Editor's Note: In 1999, the U.S. manufacturer of cisapride changed product labeling to indicate that the concurrent use of grapefruit juice and cisapride are contraindicated due to potential increases in cisapride plasma concentrations and an increased risk of ADRs.

Kivisto KT et al (Neuvonen PJ, Dept Clin Pharmacol, Univ Helsinki, Haartmaninkatu 4, FIN-00290 Helsinki, Finland; e-mail:pertti.neuvonen@huch.fi) Repeated consumption of grapefruit juice considerably increases plasma concentrations of cisapride. Clin Pharmacol & Ther 66:448–453 (Nov) 1999

CISAPRIDE
QTc Prolongation, FDA Advisory, Dear Health Professional Letter

On January 24, 2000 the manufacturer of cisapride (Janssen Pharmaceuticals) contacted health professionals regarding postmarketing adverse events, specifically QT prolongation and serious cardiac arrhythmias. The manufacturer has now recommended that a 12-lead electrocardiogram be obtained prior to cisapride initiation, that this agent should not be started if the QTc interval is greater than 450 milliseconds, and that cisapride is contraindicated in patients with electrolyte disorders. It was also recommended that serum electrolytes be monitored in diuretic treated patients prior to the initiation of cisapride therapy and periodically thereafter. This information is based on serious cardiac arrhythmias, Torsades de pointes and QT prolongation in more than 270 spontaneous reports, which included 70 deaths. The majority of these events occurred in patients at risk. In addition, health care professionals were encouraged to report serious adverse events to the manufacturer and the FDA MedWatch program.

Important safety information—propulsid health professional letter. Janssen Pharmaceuticals (Jan 24) 2000. (http://www.fda.gov/medwatch/safety/2000/propul.htm)

CISAPRIDE
Market Withdrawal due to Adverse Events

On March 23, 2000 the manufacturer of cisapride (Janssen Pharmaceuticals) notified health professionals that the company would stop manufacturing cisapride in the United States as of July 14th, 2000. As of December 31st, 1999 cisapride use has been associated with approximately 341 reports of cardiac rhythm irregularities, including 80 deaths. An earlier edition of Clin Alert (Feb 15, 2000) discusses previous FDA and manufacturer notifications regarding these cardiac abnormalities. The majority of these events occurred in patients at risk, including those with underlying conditions and/or taking other medications known to increase the risk of cardiac arrhythmias. Early notification of the pending market withdrawal was intended to provide sufficient time to determine alternative therapies. In addition, health care professionals are encouraged to report serious adverse events to the manufacturer and the FDA MedWatch program.

Janssen Pharmaceuticals stops marketing cisapride in the United States (Mar 23) 2000. (http://www.fda.gov/bbs/topics/ANSWERS/ANS01007.html) JAMA 283(21):2822–2825 (Jun 7) 2000

INFLIXIMAB
Possible Increased Susceptibility to Listeriosis
(First Report*)

A 67-year-old patient with Crohn's disease was hospitalized for weakness, lethargy, rigors, diarrhea and fever, which developed within four days after his third treatment course of infliximab. Dosages for this therapy were not provided. Other concurrent medications included oral prednisone (40 mg daily), azathioprine (150 mg daily), and mesalamine (750 mg three times daily). The patient also admitted to eating processed meats during the week prior to admission. Although symptoms and fever subsided after two days of intravenous antibiotic therapy, initial blood cultures revealed Listeria monocytogenes. The patient was continued on amoxicillin/clavulanate (750 mg twice daily for two weeks) after discharge from the hospital.

The authors noted that this is the first report of *Listeria monocytogenes* in a Crohn's patient being treated with infliximab. Although an exact mechanism of action is not clear, the authors proposed that infliximab's immunosuppressive activity may have allowed the development of infection in this patient.

Morelli J & Wilson FA (Div Gastroenterology & Hepatology, Med Univ South Carolina, Charleston, SC) Does administration of infliximab increase susceptibility to Listeriosis? Am J Gastroenterol 95(3):841–832 (Mar) 2000 (letter)

MISOPROSTOL
FDA Advisory: Contraindication in Pregnancy, Abortion

On August 23, 2000, the manufacturer of misoprostol (Searle) and the FDA reminded health professionals that the off-label use of misoprostol in pregnant women is contraindicated because it can cause abortion. Misoprostol is not FDA approved in the United States for cervical ripening in labor induction or abortion. Postmarketing data have been reported regarding serious events when the drug was used for these off-label indications, including maternal or fetal death, uterine hyperstimulation, uterine rupture/perforation, amniotic fluid embolism, severe vaginal bleeding, retained placenta, fetal bradycardia, shock, and/or pelvic pain. In the United States, misoprostol is FDA approved for the prevention of NSAID induced gastric ulcers in high-risk patients. The pharmaceutical manufacturer also announced that the company does not intend to study these off-labeled uses.

Important drug warning concerning unapproved use of intravaginal or oral misoprostol in pregnant women for induction of labor or abortion. (Aug 23) 2000. http://www.fda.gov/medwatch/safety/2000/cytote.htm

OMEPRAZOLE AND CLARITHROMYCIN
Interaction: Omeprazole Concentrations Increased

In a double blinded, randomized cross-over study, 21 healthy volunteers received either placebo or clarithromycin (400 mg twice daily) for three days followed by a morning dose of omeprazole (20 mg) with clarithromycin (400 mg) or placebo. CYP 2C19 genotype status was determined, with six subjects classified as homozygous extensive metabolizers, 11 subjects classified as heterozygous extensive metabolizers and four subjects as poor metabolizers. In all groups, plasma omeprazole levels were significantly increased (greater than two fold) during concurrent clarithromycin administration. AUC omeprazole values were highest in the poor metabolizer group (13,098.6 ng/hr/mL) as compared to the heterozygous extensive metabolizers (2,110.4 ng/hr/mL) and homozygous extensive metabolizers (813.1 ng/hr/mL). Mean AUC values for omeprazole-sulfone (a metabolite of omeprazole via CYP3A4 isoenzyme) were also highest in the poor metabolizer group when compared to the two extensive metabolizer groups (3,304.2 vs 435.3 vs 188.6). In contrast, AUC mean values for 5-hydroxy omeprazole were lowest in the poor metabolizer group (220.5 vs 1016.8 vs 946.0).

The authors concluded that omeprazole increased plasma concentrations of clarithromycin in all genotypes groups, but caused greater increases in the CYP2C19 poor metabolizer group. They also suggested that the combination use of these agents to treat H. pylori ulcers may result in higher eradication rates because of increased plasma levels.

Furuta T et al (First Dept of Med, Hamamatsu Uni Sch Med, 3600, Handa-cho, Hamamatsu, 431-3192, Japan) Effects of clarithromycin on the metabolism of omeprazole in relation to CYP2C19 genotype status in humans. Clin Pharmacol & Ther 66:265–274 (Sep) 1999

OMEPRAZOLE
Interstitial Nephritis

A 78-year-old woman was hospitalized with acute renal failure approximately two weeks after starting omeprazole for dysphagia (no dosage provided). Initial elevated laboratory values included blood urea nitrogen (45 mg/dL), serum creatinine (3.9 mg/dL), and white blood cell count (13,100/mm 3 with 15% eosinophils). Because of proteinuria and pyuria, she was treated with antibiotics for a suspected urinary tract infection. However, when BUN and serum creatinine continued to increase (58 mg/dL and 5.5 mg/dL, respectively), she was hospitalized. Other laboratory values and serum markers were within normal ranges. Because of the temporal relationship between omeprazole administration and symptom appearance a diagnosis of omeprazole induced acute interstitial nephritis was suggested and omeprazole therapy was discontinued. Serum creatinine values decreased to 2.8 mg/dL within one week and 1.4 mg/dL within two weeks after the drug was stopped.

The authors concluded that omeprazole was responsible for acute interstitial nephritis in this patient. An exact mechanism of action was not provided.

Geetha D (Div Renal Med, Johns Hopkins Bayview Med Center, Baltimore, MD 21224) Omeprazole induced acute interstitial nephritis. Am J Gastroenterol 94(11):3375–3376 (Nov) 1999 (letter)

ONDANSETRON
Acute Myocardial Infarction

A 60-year-old post-operative inpatient developed severe substernal chest pain and hypertension (158/70 mmHg) immediately after receiving an intravenous injection of ondansetron (2 mg) for refractory post-operative nausea. Previous therapy with three doses of intravenous droperidol (0.625 mg 30 minutes apart) was unsuccessful. Pain relief was achieved with epidural ropivacaine and fentanyl. Continuous electrocardiogram monitoring prior to ondansetron was unremarkable but revealed marked ST depression in the inferolateral leads after ondansetron administration. Other signs included ventricular and supraventricular tachyarrhythmias with a ventricular rate of 178 beats/minute. Symptoms resolved after sublingual nitroglycerin was administered (0.4 mg). Subsequent ECGs were not different from preoperative readings. The remainder of the hospital course was uneventful and the patient was discharged. Post-discharge cardiac evaluation found no evidence of ischemia or anatomical abnormalities.

The authors concluded that this patient's symptoms were most likely ondansetron induced myocardial ischemia. They suggested that ondansetron may suppress 5-HT3 cardiac receptors, possibly inhibiting Bezold-Jarisch reflex, causing tachyarrhythmias and possibly leading to coronary vasoconstriction.

Bosek V et al (Dept Anesthesiology, H Lee Moffitt Cancer Center, 12902 Magnolia Dr, Tampa, FL 33612-9497; e-mail:bosekv@moffitt.usf.edu) Acute myocardial ischemia after administration of ondansetron hydrochloride. Anesthesiology 92(3):885–887 (Mar) 2000

PHOSPHATE ENEMA
Hypocalcemia (Infant)

A six-week premature infant was hospitalized for apnea, and generalized seizures within 24 hours after the parent administered a full pediatric phosphate enema for suspected constipation. The only concurrent product was regular infant formula. Other symptoms and signs upon admission included bradycardia, lethargy, and frequent limb spasms. Treatment included cardiopulmonary resuscitation, epinephrine, sodium bicarbonate (3 mEq/kg), phenobarbital, and cefotaxime (for suspected infection). Screenings for infectious etiologies were negative. Abnormal laboratory values included elevated serum phosphorus (28.5 mg/dL), elevated intact serum parathyroid hormone (137 pg/mL), decreased serum calcium (2.4 mg/dL), and decreased magnesium (1 mg/dL). Intravenous bolus doses of magnesium and calcium resulted in normal serum values by day four. After 12 days of hospitalization, the patient was discharged under the care of a relative.

The authors concluded that this near fatal electrolyte disturbance was associated with the use of a nonprescription enema product. They suggested that proper management of constipation should be discussed with new parents to avoid such dangerous scenarios.

Walton DM et al (Aly MZ, Dept Neonatology, Children's Nat Med Center, 111 Michigan Ave, Washington, DC, 20010; e-mail: haly@cnmc.org) Morbid hypocalcemia associated with phosphate enema in a six-week-old infant. Pediatrics 106(3):e37–e38 (Sep) 2000

PROCHLORPERAZINE
Akathisia

In a prospective case controlled study, 100 adult patients (mean age: 31 yrs) receiving intravenous prochlorperazine (10 mg over two minutes) during an emergency room visit for severe headache or vomiting were matched to 40 control patients (mean age: 29 yrs) who received saline solutions or antibiotics. Patients were excluded if they had pre-existing motor disorders or had recently received a medication with extrapyramidal, anticholinergic, sedative or akathisia properties. The incidence of prochlorperazine induced akathisia within one hour after administration was 44% in the study group and 0% in the control group. Of the akathisia cases, 14 were rated as mild, 22 as moderate and eight as severe. Only three of 62 evaluable patients developed subjective symptoms of mild akathisia 48 hours after receiving the medication, indicating that delayed symptoms are not commonly a problem.

The authors concluded that anti-emetic induced akathisia is a common problem in the practice setting. They suggested that further research is needed to identify methods for preventing akathisia (e.g., adjuvant diphenhydramine).

Drotts DL & Vinson DR (D. Vinson, Dept of Emerg Med, Kaiser Permanente Med Center, 2025 Morse Ave, Sacramento, CA 95825) Prochlorperazine induces akathisia in emergency patients. Ann Emerg Med 34(4):469–475 (Oct) 1999

PROTON PUMP INHIBITORS
Anaphylactic Reactions

Two cases of anaphylactic reactions are described in two adult patients.

Patient 1: A 51-year-old patient developed periorbital edema, pruritis, nausea and vomiting within 45 minutes after taking the first dose of omeprazole (40 mg). There were no concurrent medications. Symptoms resolved with intravenous clemastine. A medication history revealed that the patient had previously taken the drug without event. Rechallenge with lansoprazole (30 mg) in a supervised setting resulted in more serious symptoms, including loss of consciousness, urticaria, and facial edema. Symptoms also responded to intravenous clemastine (2 mg).

Patient 2: A 62-year-old man developed malaise, hypotension (75/50 mmHg), tremors, urticaria, tongue and ocular edema within hours after taking one dose of pantoprazole. Concurrent medications included metoprolol, lisinopril, and isosorbide dinitrate (no dosages provided). A medication history revealed that the patient had taken this proton pump inhibitor within the previous year without event. Although symptoms resolved after treatment with intravenous clemastine and dexamethasone, the patient was hospitalized for observation.

The authors concluded that, although these are rare reactions, chemically related proton pump inhibitors may cause anaphylaxis. Based on the information from patient case #1 they also suggested that cross reactivity between these agents may occur.

Natsch S et al (Dept Clin Pharm, Univ Hosp Nijmegen, PO Box 9101, 6500 HB Nijmegen, the Netherlands) Anaphylactic reactions to proton pump inhibitors. Ann Pharmacother 34:474–476 (Apr) 2000

PSYLLIUM
Bronchiolitis

A 48-year-old healthy woman developed a nonproductive cough within a few days after accidentally inhaling one teaspoonful of psyllium intended for ingestion for chronic constipation. Symptoms progressed to dyspnea with approximately 20% reduction in lung diffusion capacity. Chest x-rays revealed a bibasalir, nodular interstitial abnormality at the base of both lungs. Bronchoscopy revealed normal airways and cultures of lung washings were negative. A thoracoscopic lung biopsy was performed one-month post inhalation event due to symptom persistence. These results indicated a granulomatous inflammatory process in the small airways and respiratory bronchioles. Treatment included steroids (tapered over one month) and bronchodilators, which improved symptoms and lung function.

The authors concluded that psyllium aspiration caused a granulomatous bronchiolitis and foreign body reaction in this patient.

Janoski MM et al (Barrie JR, Dept Radiology & Diagnostic Imaging, Div Thoracic Imaging, Univ Alberta Hosp, 8440-112 St, Edmonton, Alberta T6G 2B7 Canada) Psyllium aspiration causing bronchiolitis: Radiographic high resolution CT, and pathologic findings. AJR 174:799–801 (Mar) 2000

RANITIDINE
Toxic Epidermal Necrolysis (Second Case Report*)

A 31-year-old with idiopathic thrombocytopenia purpura developed erythematous macules on the trunk within one week after starting oral deflazacort (105 mg daily) and ranitidine (150 mg twice daily). Skin sloughing developed over large areas of skin and toxic epidermal necrolysis was diagnosed based on skin biopsy. Ranitidine therapy was stopped. Treatment included support therapy in a burn unit and topical mupirocin and oral ciprofloxacin. An uneventful recovery occurred over a three week period.

The authors noted that this was only the second case report of ranitidine induced toxic epidermal necrolysis and that both cases were in patients with idiopathic thrombocytopenia purpura. Although a mechanism of action was not provided, they recommended that clinicians use caution when prescribing ranitidine in patients with idiopathic thrombocytopenia purpura.

Velez A & Moreno JC (Sect Dermatol, Hosp Univ Reina Sofia, 14004 Cordoba, Spain) Second case of ranitidine related toxic epidermal necrolysis in a patient with idiopathic thrombocytopenia purpura. J Am Acad Dermatol 42(2):305 (Feb) 2000 (letter)

SULFASALAZINE
Immune Complex Hemolytic Anemia

A 79-year-old patient was hospitalized for hemolytic anemia. Medications upon admission included chronic sulfasalazine (five years), digoxin, verapamil, aspirin and oxazepam. Hemoglobin upon admission was 8.2 g/dL. The aspirin, sulfasalazine and oxazepam were discontinued upon admission and two units of blood were administered. Rechallenge with sulfasalazine resulted in another decrease in hemoglobin and increases in lactate dehydrogenase (2620 U/L) and total bilirubin (1.4 mg/dL). However, these values returned to baseline after sulfasalazine was withdrawn. The patient had normal concentrations of glucose-6-phosphate dehydrogenase and a lack of Heinz bodies on blood smear.

The authors suggested that this patient experienced immune complex hemolytic anemia as a result of sulfasalazine therapy. They also noted that a small percentage of patients with ulcerative colitis not receiving sulfasalazine will develop immune hemolytic anemia (1.7%).

Teplitsky V et al (Dept Intern Med E, Hematological Instit, Wolfson Med Center, Tel Aviv Univ, Israel) Immune complex hemolytic anemia associated with sulfasalazine. Br Med J 320:1113 (Apr 22) 2000 (letter)

HORMONES
HORMONES
HORMONES
HORMONES
HORMONES
HORMONES

Drug	Interacting Drug	ADR	Page Number
Diabetic Agents			
Glimperide		Thrombocytopenic purpura*	167
Glyburide	Ciprofloxacin	Hypoglycemia (resistant)	167
Metformin		Hemolytic anemia	168
Rosiglitazone		Hepatotoxicity	169
Troglitazone		Rheumatoid arthritis exacerbation	169
Troglitazone		Market withdrawal due to ADRs	170
Estrogens and Miscellaneous			
Clomiphene		Hypertriglyceridemia	170
Contraceptives (oral)		Pulmonary embolism^	171
Contraceptives (oral)		Ischemic stroke	171
Diethylstibesterol		Gynecologic cancer rate post in utero exposure	172
Estrogen		Melasma	174
Estrogen (topical)		Prepubertal gynecomastia (indirect exposure)	172
Steroids (Anabolic, Androgenic, Corticosteroids)			
Anabolic steroids		Renal cell carcinoma*	174
Methylprednisolone	Antiretroviral	Immunosuppression(+)	175
Methylprednisolone	Grapefruit juice	Methylprednisolone concentrations increased	175
Prednisone		Hip necrosis, med error (+)	176
Prednisone		Osteonecrosis (+)	176
Triamcinolone		Infection, scarring (+)	177
Thyroid Agents			
Levothyroxine	Calcium carbonate	Levothyroxine absorption reduced	177

Drug	Interacting Drug	ADR	Page Number
Propylthiouracil		Disseminated intravascular coagulation*	178
Thyroxine		Intolerance in iron deficiency anemia	178

* = first report
^ = death
(+) = legal action

Hormones

DIABETIC AGENTS
GLIMEPIRIDE
Thrombocytopenic Purpura (First Report*)

A 68-year-old man was hospitalized for petechial rash on the trunk, legs and face accompanied by bullae in gingival bleeding. These effects occurred approximately two months after glimepiride was started (1 mg daily). Other concurrent medications included pipotiazine (12.5 mg every six weeks), and trihexyphenidyl (4 mg daily). Glimepiride was stopped for a short period of time (less than two weeks). When restarted the patient developed hemorrhagic syndrome marked by thrombocytopenia (1×10/L). A bone marrow biopsy was negative for infectious processes, as were other tests for viral or bacterial etiologies. All medications were stopped and treatment included prednisone (1 mg/kg/day) and immunoglobulins (0.4 g/kg/day). The hemorrhagic syndrome improved by one week but the platelet count did not return to baseline until after four weeks of prednisone therapy. At six months the platelet count was still normal.

The authors concluded that this report was the first published case of glimepiride associated thrombocytopenic purpura. No mechanism of action was provided. They also recommended that platelet counts should be monitored when hemorrhagic syndrome occurs in patients taking glimepiride.

Cartron G et al (Dept Med Oncol, Bretonneau Hosp, 37 044 Tours, France) Glimepiride induced thrombocytopenic purpura. Ann Pharmacotherapy 34:120 (Jan) 2000 (letter)

GLYBURIDE AND CIPROFLOXACIN
Interaction: Resistant Hypoglycemia

An 89-year-old nursing home resident became confused and developed slurred speech and diaphoresis approximately seven days after starting ciprofloxacin (250 mg twice daily) for acute cystitis. Chronic medications included glyburide (5 mg daily), lansoprazole (15 mg twice daily), calcitonin nasal spray (200 mcg daily), celecoxib (100 mg twice daily), docusate sodium (100 mg twice daily), senna/docusate sodium (twice daily), and citalopram (20 mg daily). Upon hospital admission, serum glucose was low (57 mg/dL) but other signs and symptoms (pulse, blood pressure, urinalysis, temperature) were within normal ranges. After ingestion of orange juice with two sugar packets, serum glucose remained low (41 mg/dL) indicating resistant hypoglycemia. Treatment included intravenous 10% dextrose and oral alimentation to maintain normal glucose levels. Serum glyburide levels were 1050 ng/mL.

The authors suggested that the addition of ciprofloxacin to this patient's stable drug regimen was responsible for the development of resistant hypoglycemia. They proposed that elevated glyburide levels were induced via ciprofloxacin inhibition of P-450 CYP3A4 isoenzymes, and suggested that close patient monitoring is warranted during combination therapy.

Roberge RJ et al (Kaplan R, Dept Emergency Med, Western Pennsylvania Hosp, 4800 Friendship Ave, Pittsburgh, PA 15224) Glyburide-ciprofloxacin interaction with resistant hypoglycemia. Ann Emerg Med 36(2):160–163 (Aug) 2000

METFORMIN
Hemolytic Anemia (Second Report*)

A 51-year-old newly diagnosed diabetic developed fatigue and jaundice approximately nine days after starting metformin therapy (850 mg twice daily). Investigative laboratory tests suggested a hemolytic anemia via a reduced hemoglobin (9.1 g/dL) and hematocrit (0.30) accompanied by an increased mean corpuscular volume (102 fl) and reticulocyte count (0.045%). However, platelet and leukocyte counts were within normal ranges. Liver function tests were also within normal ranges but other increased tests included plasma lactate dehydrogenase (300 IU), serum total bilirubin (112 umol/L) and unconjugated bilirubin (85 umol/L). Viral and bacteriological etiologies for jaundice or liver involvement were negative. Within six weeks after metformin was discontinued, jaundice resolved and bilirubin values returned to baseline. Rechallenge with metformin (500 mg daily) resulted in return of fatigue and scleral icterus by the third day of therapy. Serum total bilirubin and unconjugated fraction were 59 umol/L and 42 umol/L, respectively. Post drug withdrawal serum bilirubin returned to baseline within 12 days.

The authors concluded that metformin was responsible for hemolytic anemia in this patient also resulting in jaundice and hyperbilirubinemia. They also noted that this is only the second published report of this adverse effect attributed to the drug. Health care practitioners should be aware of this potential complication.

Kashyap AS & Kashyap S (Dept Med, Armed Forces Med Coll, Pune 411040, India) Haemolytic anemia due to metformin. Postgrad Med J 76:125–126 (Feb) 2000

ROSIGLITAZONE
Hepatotoxicity

A 61-year-old man with type II diabetes was hospitalized for jaundice approximately two weeks after starting rosiglitazone therapy (4 mg daily). Symptoms started approximately eight days after therapy was initiated. Other chronic medications included bronchodilators, theophylline, prednisone and zafirlukast (no dosages provided). The patient also used acetaminophen (three to four tablets daily) on a chronic basis for three months prior to admission. Upon admission, liver function tests and related laboratory values were elevated including, total bilirubin (9.6 mg/dL), direct bilirubin (8.7 mg/dL), alkaline phosphatase (331 U/L), aspartate aminotransferase (1370 U/L), alanine aminotransferase (1706 U/L) and gamma glutamyltransferase (14.64 U/L). Bacterial and viral etiologies were ruled out. Acetaminophen serum levels were below normal therapeutic limits (3.2 mcg/mL). Rosiglitazone therapy was discontinued upon hospitalization and by the second day symptoms resolved. However, liver enzymes slowly decreased over eight days with subsequent discharge. All liver function tests were within normal ranges at a follow-up seven weeks later.

The authors suggested that rosiglitazone was the most likely cause of hepatotoxicity in this patient. Because rosiglitazone occurred earlier than the manufacturer recommended monitoring guidelines (every two months), the authors suggested earlier monitoring after initiation of therapy. Specifically, they suggested weekly for the first two to four weeks and monthly thereafter for the first year.

Al-Salman J et al (Mittal MK: Div Gastroenterol, Easton Hosp, 250 South 21st St, Easton, PA 18042) Hepatocellular injury in a patient receiving rosiglitazone. Ann Intern Med 132:121–124 (Jan 18) 2000

TROGLITAZONE
Deterioration of Rheumatoid Arthritis

A 49-year-old woman with rheumatoid arthritis and diabetes developed severe joint pain in the elbows, fingers and krees several days after adding troglitazone (400 mg daily) to her diabetic regimen. Two days after stopping the troglitazone her joint pain improved. Other medications included ketoprofen (75 mg daily), oxaprozin (400 mg daily), prednisolone (5 mg daily), glyburide (7.5 mg daily) and acarbose (300 mg daily). Rechallenge with troglitazone occurred five months later resulting in recurring joint pain which again resolved upon drug withdrawal. However, during this time, no changes occurred in rheumatoid arthritis testing, including C-reactive protein, rheumatoid factor or erythrocyte sedimentation rates. Based on the temporal association between the administration of troglitazone and appearance/disappearance of symptoms, the authors concluded that troglitazone most likely precipitated joint pain in this patient. A clear mechanism of action has not been established, but the authors suggested that clinicians carefully monitor symptoms of arthritis patients during troglitazone therapy.

Sakurai A & Hashizume K (Dept Aging Med & Geriatrics, Shinshu Univ Sch Med, Matsumoto, Japan) Deterioration of rheumatoid arthritis with troglitazone: a rare and unexpected adverse effect. Arch Intern Med 160:118–119 (Jan 10) 2000 (letter)

TROGLITAZONE
Market Withdrawal Due to Adverse Events

On March 21, 2000 the manufacturer of troglitazone (Parke Davis/ Warner Lambert) notified health professionals that the company would stop manufacturing the product. As of 1997 troglitazone use has been associated with severe hepatotoxicity and in some cases, resulting in death. Previous FDA and manufacturer notifications have been published regarding increased monitoring of liver function during troglitazone therapy. The availability of two newer and similar drugs with less risk of severe liver toxicity contributed to the decision of market withdrawal of troglitazone. In addition, health care professionals are encouraged to report serious adverse events to the manufacturer and the FDA MedWatch program.

Rezulin to be withdrawn from the market (Mar 21) 2000. (http://www.fda.gov/bbs/topics/ NEWS/NEW00721.html)

ESTROGENS AND MISCELLANEOUS
CLOMIPHENE
Hypertriglyceridemia

A 37-year-old woman developed severe abdominal pain, nausea, vomiting and fever within two months of starting clomiphene (50 mg to 150 mg daily over two months). Laboratory testing revealed an elevated white blood cell count (19.0 × 10/L), cholesterol (222 mg/dL) and triglycerides (570 mg/dL). Liver function tests, amylases and lipases, however, were within normal ranges. Abdominal scans indicated a fatty infiltrate of the liver and pancreatic edema. Symptoms resolved after clomiphene was stopped. A similar episode recurred after clomiphene was restarted (150 mg to 200 mg daily) with elevated levels for amylase (410 U/L), lipase (3320 U/L), total cholesterol (609 mg/dL) and triglycerides (5314 mg/dL). Clomiphene was discontinued. And within three weeks of starting gemfibrozil therapy total cholesterol and triglycerides were reduced and amylase and lipase levels had normalized.

The authors recommended that women with a history of hypertriglyceridemia should have baseline lipid levels determined prior to clomiphene therapy.

Castro MR et al (O'Brien T: Div Endocrinology, Metabolism & Nutrition, Mayo Clinic, Rochester, 200 First St SW, Rochester, MN 55905) Clomiphene induced severe hypertriglyceridemia and pancreatitis. Mayo Clin Proc 74:1125–1128 (Nov) 1999

ORAL CONTRACEPTIVES
Fatal Pulmonary Embolism

In a retrospective case control study, the risk of fatal pulmonary embolism was studied in New Zealand women (aged 15 to 49 years) who used combined oral contraceptives. Twenty six contraceptive users (median age: 29 yrs) who died of pulmonary embolism were compared to 111 control patients. When compared to nonusers of any combined oral contraceptives, the odds ratio for pulmonary embolism in current users of all types of contraceptives was 9.6. Of the women who died from pulmonary embolism during contraceptive therapy, only three were first time users of any combined product. The most commonly used products by the case group included desogestrel (seven) or gestodene (five). Two cases, on cyproterone acetate and ethinylestradiol, had a risk ratio of 17.6.

The authors concluded that in this case control study the risk of fatal pulmonary embolism was increased in women who used oral contraceptives. They also noted that although death from pulmonary embolism is rare in oral contraceptive users, this information indicates that this complication remains clinically important.

Parkin L et al (Skegg DCG, Dept Preventive Med & Social Med, Univ Ottago, PO Box 913, Dunedin, New Zealand) Oral contraceptives and fatal pulmonary embolism. Lancet 355:2133–2134 (Jun 17) 2000

ORAL CONTRACEPTIVES
Ischemic Stroke

A meta-analysis of 16 studies evaluated the risk of ischemic stroke associated with the use of oral contraceptives. The overall summary risk estimated for ischemic stroke was 2.75 for current oral contraceptive users compared to non-users (currently). This relative risk was significant in 11 of the 16 studies. An increased risk of ischemic stroke was lower but still significantly elevated with reduced estrogen doses (<50 mcg) when compared to high estrogen doses (>50 mcg), producing relative risks of 2.08 vs 4.53, respectively. Lower risks were also found in studies using low estrogen products and controlling for both smoking and hypertension (relative risk: 1.93). When this data is extrapolated, it is estimated that

4.1 ischemic strokes would occur per 100,000 nonsmoking, normotensive women who use low-estrogen oral contraceptives or one additional ischemic stroke/year/24,000 women. The authors concluded that although the risk of ischemic stroke is increased in women who currently use oral contraceptives, the incidence of this potential complication remains low.

Gillum LA et al (Johnston SC:Dept Neurology, Box 0114, Univ California, San Francisco, 505 Parnassus Ave, San Franscisco, CA 94143-0114; e-mail:clayj@itsa.ucsf.edu) Ishemic stroke risk with oral contraceptives. A meta-analysis. JAMA 284:72–78 (Jul 5) 2000

DIETHYLSTIBESTEROL
Prevalence of Gynecologic Cancer In Women Exposed in Utero

A questionnaire mailed to 13,350 women exposed to diethylstibesterol in utero assessed self-reported data on cancer rates in this population and compared it to expected rates. Cancer information reported by patients was verified by medical record documentation. Approximately 41% response rate was recorded with a median age of the respondents being 30 years of age. The age range for the respondents was 19 to 45 years. A total of 111 cancers were reported by 105 women. Medical records were reviewed and confirmed in 85 patients. The prevalence ratio for only cervical cancer was significantly higher in diethylstibesterol-exposed women than expected in the general population (5.4 vs 2.22). Other cancers assessed included vulva, breast, ovarian, melanoma, and colon.

Based on these results, the authors suggested that cervical cancer rates are higher in women who have been exposed to diethylstibesterol in utero. However, they also noted that the results may have been influenced by the fact that women with health problems were more likely to complete the survey. The authors suggested that larger studies are required to validate these initial observations.

Verloop J et al (Netherlands Cancer Instit, 1066 CX Amsterdam, the Netherlands) Prevalence of gynecologic cancer in women exposed to diethylstibesterol in utero. N Engl J Med 342(24):1837–1838 (Jun 15) 2000 (letter)

ESTROGEN CREAM
Prepubertal Gynecomastia after Indirect Exposure (First Reports*)

Three cases of prepubertal gynecomastia are described in prepubertal boys (age range: 28 months to 8 yrs) who were indirectly exposed to estrogen cream used by their mothers.

Patient #1: A 33-month-old boy developed bilateral breast enlargement and a rapid growth increase over a six month period. No medications were taken during this time period and the patient had an otherwise normal developmental history. In addition, there was no familial history of gynecomastia or early puberty. Physical examination revealed Tanner II breast development with 2 cm of glandular breast tissue bilaterally. Other pubertal development was not apparent (i.e., pubic or axillary hair, acne, penile enlargement). Assessment six months later documented continued increased growth patterns and breast enlargement and elevated estradiol levels (3.5 ng/dL). It was discovered that the mother was applying a compounded topical estrogen cream (9 mg estradiol/1 gm cream) twice daily to her thighs. Four months after the mother switched to a transdermal estrogen patch, the child's estradiol level returned to normal (0.6 ng/mL) and breast tissue had decreased. At 4.25 yrs the child's bone age was 8 yrs and 10 months. During a 2 year follow-up period, gynecomastia did not recur.

Patient #2: A 28-month-old boy developed bilateral breast enlargement and rapid growth increase. No medications were taken during this time period. The mother was applying a compounded topical estrogen cream (9 mg estradiol/1 gm cream) twice daily to her thighs for the previous eight months. Physical examination revealed Tanner II-III breast development with 2.5 cm of glandular breast tissue bilaterally. Estradiol levels were elevated (4.8 ng/dL). Other pubertal development was not apparent. Six months after the mother discontinued the use of estrogen cream, breast size had decreased significantly and estradiol levels were undetectable (<0.5 ng/dL). During a 16 month follow-up period, gynecomastia did not recur.

Patient #3: An 8-year-old boy developed bilateral breast enlargement. Chronic medication included methylphenidate (twice daily) for the last two years. The mother was applying a compounded topical estrogen cream (24 mg estradiol/1 gm cream) twice daily to her abdomen for the previous four months. Physical examination revealed Tanner II breast development with 1.5 to 2 cm of glandular breast tissue bilaterally. Estradiol levels were elevated (10 ng/dL). Other pubertal development was not apparent. Four months after the mother discontinued the use of estrogen cream, breast size had decreased significantly and estradiol levels were undetectable (<0.5 ng/dL). During a one year follow-up period, gynecomastia did not recur.

The authors concluded that these boys developed gynecomastia as a result of indirect exposure to estrogen products that the mothers were using. The authors suggested that the most likely routes of transmission were via the mothers' hands after topical application or possibly via food preparation. Clinicians should consider the possibility of indirect estrogen exposure when examining prepubertal boys with gynecomastia.

Felner EI & White PC (Depts Pediatrics & Endocrinology, 5323 Harry Hines Blvd, Dallas TX 75235; e-mail:efelne@childmed.dallas.tx.us) Prepubertal gynecomastia: indirect exposure to estrogen cream. Pediatrics 105(4):e55–57 (Apr) 2000 (http://www.pediatrics.org/cgi/content/full/105/4/e55)

ESTROGEN/PROGESTIN REPLACEMENT
Melasma

A 46-year-old woman developed bilateral and irregular pigmentation of both forearms after sun exposure during chronic estrogen/progestin hormone replacement therapy (estradiol valerate 2 mg and levonorgestrel 75 mcg once daily). The patient reported sunscreen use on both her face (SPF 12) and arms (SPF 6) and no history of previous skin diseases. The pigmentation gradually faded over a 16-week period after switching to another product containing estradiol 1 mg and dydrogesterone 10 mg.

The authors concluded that ultraviolet radiation from the sun and hormonally induced melanocyte in the skin may interact to cause hyperpigmentation. The use of a higher SPF factor sunscreen on the face in this patient may have prevented facial pigmentation. The authors advised that patients should be counseled to protect their skin from sun-exposure and to use sunscreens when taking hormone replacement.

Varma S & Roberts DL (Dept Dermatol, Univ Hosp Wales, Heath Park, Cardiff CF4 4XW, U.K) Melasma of the arms associated with hormone replacement therapy. Br J Dermatol 141:592 (Sep) 1999 (letter)

STEROIDS *(Anabolic, Androgenic, Corticosteroid)*
ANABOLIC STEROIDS
Renal Cell Carcinoma (Second Report*)

A 39-year-old man who abused anabolic steroids for 15 years developed renal cell carcinoma. Anabolic steroid use included testosterone propionate (two week cycles), mixed testosterone esters (16 week cycles), stanozolol (24 week cycles), and methenolone (16 week cycles). Although a physical examination was normal, the patient had experienced significant recent weight loss. An abdominal ultrasound and CT scan revealed a large mass on the right kidney. A right nephrectomy, adrenalectomy and lymphadenectomy were performed. Histological examination of the removed tissue revealed renal cell adenocarcinoma.

The authors noted that this publication is only the second case report of renal cell carcinoma associated with anabolic steroid use. Although anabolic androgen use and cancers of other organs (liver and prostate) have been reported, renal carcinomas have only been linked to steroid use in animals. The authors suggested that exogenous androgens might promote renal hypertrophy and malignant growth. They also recommended that this potential hazard should be promoted to sports organizations to educate body builders about the hazards of steroid use and to prevent potential complications associated with steroid abuses.

Martorana G et al (Dept Urology, Univ Bologna, Policlinico S. Orsola-Malpighi, Bologna, Italy) Anabolic steroid abuse and renal cell carcinoma. J Urology 162: 2089–2090 (Dec) 1999

METHYLPREDNISOLONE AND GRAPEFRUIT JUICE
Interaction: Increased Methylprednisolone Concentrations

In a two phase, crossover study, 10 healthy subjects were randomized to receive either double strength grapefruit juice (200 mL) or water (200 mL) three times daily for two days. Oral methylprednisolone (16 mg) was administered on day three in both groups. Additional water or grapefruit juice was also ingested one half hour before and 1.5 hours after methylprednisolone administration. A washout period of four weeks was employed between study phases. Grapefruit juice slightly delayed the absorption of methylprednisolone with the time to peak concentration being significantly longer in the grapefruit juice phase (Tmax: 3.0 vs 2.0 hrs). Peak concentrations and area under the curve were also significantly higher in the grapefruit juice phase (Cmax: 128 vs 101 ng/mL; AUC: 780 vs 453 ng.hr/mL). Half-lives were also prolonged in the grapefruit juice phase (135 vs 100 hrs). However, there were no significant differences between the phases in plasma cortisol concentrations after methylprednisolone administration.

The authors concluded that grapefruit juice increased methylprednisolone plasma concentrations, most likely via CYP3A4 inhibition. Although the clinical significance of this interaction for most patients may be small, the ingestion of grapefruit juice in patients taking high doses could enhance methylprednisolone effects.

Varis T et al (Dept Clin Pharmacol, Univ Helsinki & Helsinki Univ Central Hosp, Haartmanink 4, FIN—00290 Helsinki, Finland; e-mail:pertti.neuvonen@ hus.fi) Grapefruit juice can increase the plasma concentrations of oral methylprednisolone. Eur J Clin Pharmacol 56:489–493 (Sep) 2000

METHYLPREDNISOLONE AND ANTIRETROVIRALS
Immunosuppression, Legal Action

A 39-year-old HIV positive patient received concurrent therapy with methylprednisolone (large unspecified doses), 14 HIV medications, and six diarrhea medications. Methylprednisolone doses were prescribed for a period of six months. The patient was instructed to purchase medications at a pharmacy co-owned by the prescriber. The plaintiff alleged that the chronic administration of methylprednisolone was contraindicated with concurrent HIV medications and caused immunosuppression, thus, causing the development of resistance and shortened life expectancy. A settlement of one million dollars was reached prior to the beginning of the trial.

> M Keifhaver vs LR Anisman, Pride Medical Services PC & Pride Medical, Inc. Use of steroid solumedrol for six months while taking multiple HIV medications contraindicated—weakened immune system—$1 million Georgia settlement. Med Malpractice Verdicts, Settlements & Experts 16(8):25 (Aug) 2000

PREDNISONE
Overdose, Improper Prescription Labeling, Hip Necrosis, Legal Action

A 36-year-old patient claimed that he ingested prednisone (100 mg daily) for 17 days at higher doses (50 mg vs 10 mg) instead of five days as a result of a misfilled and an improperly labeled prescription. Additional prednisone was also required for an appropriate tapering schedule. Subsequently, the patient developed avascular hip necrosis requiring bilateral hip replacements. The defendants recognized the dispensing errors but claimed that the hip necrosis was related to non-Hodgkin's lymphoma and not the prednisone overdose. A one million dollar settlement was reached during the trial.

> Oliver J & RM vs Evkin Pharm Corp, Ekstrand R & Conte V. Improper labeling of prescription—overdose of prednisone—bilateral avascular necrosis of the hips—$1 million New York Settlement. Med Malpractice, Verdicts, Settlements & Experts 16(5): 47 (May) 2000

PREDNISONE
Osteonecrosis, Legal Action

A 45-year-old patient developed osteonecrosis of the hips approximately one year after receiving two courses of prednisone for poison ivy the year before. The defendant physician initially prescribed a 10 day course of prednisone (total: 270 mg) followed by an additional 21 days (total: 750 mg) when poison ivy was unresponsive. A total of 1.02 grams was administered over approximately a one month period. The plaintiff claimed that the poison ivy was limited to the right forearm, but the defendant claimed that it extended to the face, arms, back and legs. Ultimately the hip necrosis required bilateral hip replacements. A $300,000 settlement was reached by both parties.

> Anon vs Anon Poison ivy-prednisone-osteonecrosis—$300,000 Virginia settlement. Med Malpractice Verdicts, Settlements & Experts 16(6):26 (Jun) 2000

TRIAMCINOLONE
Infection, Permanent Scarring, Legal Action

A 35-year-old patient claimed that an improper administration of triamcinolone injection into the buttocks resulted in an infected abscess requiring surgery and permanent scarring. The specific misadministration referred to failure to change needles between administering the first and second injections and improper administration into the deep intramuscular tissue. The patient was hospitalized as a result of the infection and required surgery. The defendant claimed that the injection was not responsible for the infection and that a sterile abscess is a known side effect of the drug. It was reported that the jury awarded $132,000 to the plaintiff.

O'Leary Ross K & J vs Mandel SS. Kenalog injection into buttock for psoriasis blamed for infection-surgery-permanent scarring—$132,000 New York verdict. Med Malpractice Verdicts, Settlements & Experts 16(4):8 (Apr) 2000

THYROID AGENTS
LEVOTHYROXINE AND CALCIUM CARBONATE
Interaction: T4 Absorption Reduced

In a prospective one-year cohort study, 20 adult patients with hypothyroidism stabilized on chronic levothyroxine therapy, ingested calcium carbonate (1200 mg daily of elemental calcium) for three months. At the end of three months, free T4 serum concentrations and total T4 were significantly decreased when compared to baseline (1.34 vs 1.22 ng/dL and 9.21 vs 8.55 mcg/dL). In contrast, mean thyroid stimulating hormone concentrations were significantly increased (1.6 vs 2.71 mIU/L). Mean T3 serum concentrations, however, were unchanged during concurrent administration of the two products (141.50 vs 142.10 ng/dL). All values returned to near baseline levels at two months after calcium carbonate administration was discontinued.

The authors concluded that calcium carbonate has a clinically moderate but significant impact on thyroid function. They suggested that the decrease in levothyroxine's bioavailability is mediated by levothyroxine adsorption to calcium carbonate in an acidic environment. Clinicians are advised to monitor any changes in thyroid function tests in patients who are taking both calcium carbonate and levothyroxine. Separating administration times was advised.

Singh N et al. (Div Endocrinol & Metabolism, Endocrinology 111D, VA Greater Los Angeles Healthcare System, 11301 Wilshire Blvd, Los Angeles, CA 90073; e-mail: nsingh@ucla.edu) Effect of calcium carbonate on the absorption of levothyroxine. JAMA 283(21):2822–2825 (Jun 7) 2000

PROPYLTHIOURACIL
Disseminated Intravascular Coagulation, Vasculitis (First Report*)

A 42-year-old woman was hospitalized for a purpuric rash which developed within two weeks after starting propylthiouracil for Grave's disease (100 mg three times daily). Concurrent medications were not provided or mentioned. The rash began on the face and progressed to the trunk and limbs. Abnormal laboratory tests included white blood cell count (15.5 × 10⁹/L), platelets (49 × 10⁹/L), erythrocyte sedimentation rate (23 mm/h), serum complement 4 (12 mg/dL), and elevated free thyroxine levels (3.7 ng/dL). Coagulation studies revealed a slightly elevated prothrombin time (14.3 seconds) and an activated partial prothrombin time within normal ranges (28 seconds). Urinalysis revealed hematuria and proteinuria. Skin biopsies also revealed hemorrhagic necrosis and acute inflammation. Treatment with intravenous methylprednisolone (125 mg every eight hours) resulted in gradual resolution. Steroids were tapered over a two week period.

The authors concluded that this patient's reaction was caused by propylthiouracil partially related to the involvement of the immune complex mechanism, represented by low complement serum levels. They also noted that this is the first case of propylthiouracil associated disseminated intravascular coagulation reported in an adult.

Khurshid I & Sher J (Jersey Shore Med Center, Dept Endocrinology, 1945 State Route 33, Neptune, NJ 07754) Disseminated intravascular coagulation and vasculitis during propylthiouracil therapy. Postgrad Med J 76:185–186 (Mar) 2000

THYROXINE
Intolerance in Iron Deficiency Anemia Patients

Four cases of intolerance to thyroxine therapy in women with iron deficiency anemia are described. In all cases, thyroxine was reinitiated without event after treatment with ferrous sulfate.

Patient 1: A 28-year-old patient with primary hypothyroidism and iron deficiency anemia (hematocrit: 23%) developed severe palpitations, tachycardia (120 beats per minute) and restlessness, three days after starting thyroxine sodium (50 mcg daily). Further cardiac examination revealed no abnormalities. Because symptoms persisted despite a dosage reduction (to 25 mcg daily), thyroxine was discontinued. Once the iron deficiency anemia was corrected with ferrous sulfate therapy for six weeks, the patient was able to tolerate thyroxine therapy without event. The dose was gradually increased to 112 mcg daily without further problems and thyroid function was within normal limits at a three-month follow-up.

Patient 2: A 36-year-old patient with iron deficiency anemia (hematocrit: 28%) and primary hypothyroidism developed palpitations, tachycardia (116 beats per minute) and restlessness, after five days of concurrent therapy with thyroxine sodium (25 mcg daily) and ferrous sulfate (325 mg three times daily). No other concurrent medications were taken. Further cardiac examination revealed no abnormalities. Thyroxine was discontinued. After completing seven weeks of ferrous sulfate therapy, reinitiation of thyroxine at the same dose was tolerated without event and with an eventual dosage titration to 125 mcg daily.

Patient 3: A 21-year-old patient with primary hypothyroidism and iron deficiency anemia (hematocrit: 24%) developed palpitations and tachycardia (108 beats per minute) one week after starting concurrent therapy with thyroxine sodium (25 mcg daily) and ferrous sulfate (325 mg three times daily). Further cardiac examination revealed no abnormalities. Reinitiation of thyroxine (25 mcg daily) was tolerated without event after four weeks of ferrous sulfate therapy.

Patient 4: A 33-year-old patient with iron deficiency anemia (hematocrit: 20.5%) and primary hypothyroidism developed anxiety, nervousness, and palpitations after the first dose of thyroxine sodium (50 mcg daily). Concurrent medication included ferrous sulfate (325 mg three times daily). Cardiac examination revealed no abnormalities, despite persistent symptoms during two weeks of continued thyroxine therapy. Thyroxine was discontinued. After completing six weeks of ferrous sulfate therapy, reinitiation of thyroxine was tolerated without event.

Shakir KMM et al (Endocrinology & Metabolism Div, Dept Internal Med, National Naval Med Center, Bethesda, MD 20889-5600) Anemia: a cause of intolerance to thyroxine sodium. Mayo Clin Proc 75:189–192 (Mar) 2000

VITAMINS/MINERALS
VITAMINS/MINERALS
VITAMINS/MINERALS
VITAMINS/MINERALS
VITAMINS/MINERALS
VITAMINS/MINERALS

Drug	ADR	Page Number
Vitamins/Minerals	Hypermagnesemia^	183
Zinc	Anemia, leukopenia	184
^ = death		

Vitamins/Minerals

MEGAVITAMINS/MINERALS
Fatal Hypermagnesemia

A 28-month-old boy with severe medical problems including quadriplegia and seizures, was admitted through the emergency room in cardiac arrest approximately three weeks after starting high dose vitamin and mineral supplementation per a private nutritional consultation unknown to the patient's physician. The regimen consisted of calcium carbonate, multivitamins, essential fatty acids, lactobacillus, bifodobacterium, and magnesium oxide (one-half teaspoonfuls four times daily). The dose of magnesium oxide was increased to one-half tablespoonful five times daily several days prior to admission. Symptoms prior to admission included drowsiness and difficulty arousing, progressing to unresponsiveness and dilated pupils. Upon arrival to the emergency room, cardiopulmonary resuscitation was initiated. Among the abnormal serum electrolyte values was hypermagnesemia (20.3 mg/dL) with isolated premature ventricular complexes and no p-waves on an electrocardiogram. Despite reductions in serum magnesium levels (7.6 mg/dL) via hemodialysis and supportive therapy, the patient died within 20 hours post-admission due to cardiac dysrythmias. Autopsy results included but were not limited to cardiac ischemia, bowel tissue necrosis, a calcium carbonate stone in the stomach and chalky white material in the stomach and intestines.

The authors concluded that hypermagnesemia with subsequent cardiac changes occurred in this patient as a result of a magnesium oxide overdose. They also cautioned pediatricians to inquire about alternative medicine use in order to avoid preventable adverse events.

McGuire JK et al (Div Critical Care Med, Dept Peds, St. Louis Children's Hosp, One Children's Place, St. Louis, MO 63110) Fatal hypermagnesemia in a child treated with megavitamin/megamineral therapy. Pediatrics 105(2):e18–20 (Feb) 2000. URL: http://www.pediatrics.org/cgi/reprint/105/2/e18.pdf

ZINC
Anemia, Leukopenia

A 17-year-old patient was referred for medical evaluation because of persistent refractory upper respiratory tract infections. A complete white blood count revealed exogenous bone marrow suppression and anemia, and despite the cessation of antibiotic therapy, symptoms persisted for an additional four weeks. Serologic testing for other infectious etiologies was negative. Symptoms of fatigue and fainting continued for another six months with continued low white blood cell counts and mild granulocyte hypoplasia. Serum copper and ceruloplasmin levels were decreased, less than 10 mcg/dL and 2 mg/dL, respectively. At this evaluation it was discovered that the patient had been self-medicating with a nonprescription zinc preparation (up to 300 mg daily). Serum zinc levels were above normal ranges (199 mcg/dL). Within two month after zinc supplementation was stopped, blood counts were within normal ranges and the symptoms of fatigue and headache had resolved. Follow-up evaluation at 17 months revealed normal ranges for zinc, copper and ceruloplasmin.

The authors concluded that zinc was responsible for inducing anemia and leukopenia in this patient, possibly related to the induction of a copper deficiency via increased production of metallothionein. This product is responsible for binding to copper and may result in increased copper excretion. Hypocupremia may be responsible for inducing anemia via a number of different mechanisms. The authors cautioned clinicians to be aware of this potential complication associated with high dose chronic zinc therapy.

Porea TJ et al (Texas Children's Hosp, 6621 Fannin St, MC3-3320, Houston, TX 77030) Zinc induced anemia and neutropenia in an adolescent. J Pediatr 136:688–690 (May) 2000

MISCELLANEOUS
MISCELLANEOUS
MISCELLANEOUS
MISCELLANEOUS
MISCELLANEOUS
MISCELLANEOUS

Drug	Interacting Drug	ADR	Page Number
General			
ADRs (Hepatic)		Inaccurate reporting	188
Adverse drug events		Risk factors in hospitalized patients	187
Adverse drug events		Hospital patients	187
Intravenous fluids		Phlebitis	189
Intravenous fluids		Extravasation	188
Sedation		Overdose (+)	189
Drugs			
Alendronate		Unmasked hypoparathyroidism	190
Alendronate		Hepatotoxicity	191
Alendronate		Esophageal & gastric ADRs	190
Allergy			
Immunotherapy		Anaphylactic shock^ (+)	191
Allopurinol		Hypersensitivity (familial)	192
Anesthesia		Hearing loss	192
Balsalazide		Allergy*	193
Cocaine		Hepatitis in HIV patients	193
Cocaine		Ischemic colitis	194
Cyclosporin A		Leucocytoclastic Vasculitis*	197
Cyclosporine	St. John's wort	Cyclosporine concentrations decreased	196
Donezepil		Pisa syndrome	206
Dopamine agonists		Sleep attacks	197
Etanercept		Local reactions	198
Fenfluramine		Valvular heart disease	198
Icodextrin		Allergic reactions	199
Licorice		Hypertension	200
Magnesium sulfate		Medication error	201
Orlistat		Hypertension	201
Pergolide		Sleep attacks	202
Phentermine		Valvular heart disease	198
Pramipexole		Peripheral edema	202

Drug	Interacting Drug	ADR	Page Number
Pramipexole		Sleep attacks	207
Propofol		Coughing (violent)	204
Propofol		Green urine	203
Quinine		Hemolytic uremic syndrome	204
Riluzole		Methemglobinemia (overdose)*	205
Risedronate		Esophageal & gastric ADRs	190
Rivastigmine		Pisa syndrome	206
Ropinirole		Sleep attacks	206, 207
Sildenafil		Optic neuropathy	208
Sildenafil		Priapism in sickle cell*	208
Sirolimus		Intersitial pneumonitis	209
Sodium polysterene sulfate		Colonic necoris	209
Sumatriptan		Mesenteric ischemia	210
Tacrolimus		Autoimmune diabetes	211
Temoporfin		Light exposure burns	211
Thalidomide		Toxic epidermal necrolysis*	211, 212
Trastuzumab		Serious ADRs	213
Zuclopenthixol		Neutropenia, thrombocytopenia*	213

* = first report
^ = death
(+) = legal action

Miscellaneous

GENERAL
ADVERSE DRUG EVENT (ADEs) RISK FACTORS IN HOSPITALIZED PATIENTS

In a case control study of 4108 hospital admissions, there were 190 ADEs, 60 preventable ADEs, and 84 severe ADEs (after controlled for length of stay and level of care). When compared to controls, there was no significant correlation for age, number of drugs received within 24 hours or since admission, presence of altered mental status, or presence of elevated bilirubin or creatinine levels. For all ADEs, exposure to psychoactive agents was a risk factor, as was cardiovascular drugs for severe ADEs.

The authors concluded that sicker patients with prolonged hospital stays were at increased risk of an ADE while hospitalized. They suggested that ADE prevention strategies should focus on medication system improvements rather than identifying target populations.

Bates DW et al (Div Gen Med & Primary Care, Brigham & Woman's Hosp, 75 Francis St, Boston, MA 02115; e-mail:dwbates@partners.org) Patient risk factors for adverse drug events in hospitalized patients. Arch Intern Med 159:2553–2560 (Nov 22) 1999

ADVERSE DRUG REACTIONS
Hospital Admissions

A two week prospective study of 33 French teaching and general hospitals monitored admissions related to adverse drug events. Of 3137 patients admitted, approximately 3.2% (100) were adverse drug event related. Patients admitted because of adverse drug effects were more likely to be older (greater than 65 years) and women. Gastrointestinal reactions were the most frequent drug related cause of admission, with gastrointestinal bleeding most commonly reported with nonsteroidal anti-inflammatory drugs (9). Cardiac stimulants and antiarrhythmics agents were the most frequently reported agents associated with hospitalization. (9%). Other commonly reported drugs included antineoplastics (8%), antithrombotic drugs (8%), and antihypertensives (8%). A total of 13 patients were admitted with bleeding complications due to anticoagulants. Adverse events were reversible in the majority of patients (78%) but was the direct cause of death in four patients. Mean hospital duration was 9.7 days.

The authors estimated that approximately 134,000 hospital admissions are caused by adverse events annually in France.

Pouyanne P et al (Haramburu F, Centre Reg de Pharmacovigilance Alsace, Serv de Pharmacologie Clin, Hopitaux Univ, F-67091, Strasbourg, France) Admissions to hospital caused by adverse drug reactions: cross sectional incidence study. Br Med J 320:1036 (Apr 15) 2000

HEPATIC ADVERSE DRUG REACTIONS
Inaccurate Reporting

During 1992 to 1996, 188 hepatic adverse drug reactions were reported by hospital and general practitioners in northern England to the Committee on Safety of Medicines. A total of 138 were reviewed for causality. Of these, 52 (37.7%) were considered drug-related, 65 (47.1%) were determined non-drug related, and causality could not be determined in 21 (15.2%) cases. Follow-up liver function tests in 65 patients with reactions not related to drugs indicated that the correct diagnosis was delayed in 35 cases by a median of 885 days in hospitals and by 122 days in the general practitioner groups.

The authors concluded that almost half of hepatic adverse drug reactions are likely to be unrelated to the suspected drug. They also noted that inaccurate adverse drug reaction reporting may delay needed treatment for other clinical diagnoses and may require unnecessary withdrawal of a drug. They also recommended that the diagnosis of adverse drug reactions should be based on the timing of the reaction in relation to drug administration and that diagnosis should include the exclusion of other possible causes.

Aithal GP et al (Centre for Liver Res, Med Sch, Univ of Newcastle, Newcastle upon Tyne NE2 4HH) Accuracy of hepatic adverse drug reaction re-porting in one English health region. Br Med J 319:1541 (Dec 11) 1999

INTRAVENOUS EXTRAVASATION
Hand Disfiguration

An inpatient experienced severe extravasation of an intravenous drug during a hospitalization. The plaintiff claimed that inadequate monitoring of the intravenous line and delays in stopping the infusion after complaints of discomfort contributed to the event. The patient's nondominant hand swelled to twice the normal size, resulting in full thickness skin loss. Numerous surgeries were required for skin grafting and adequate joint manipulation. The defendant nurse denied that the patient complained of discomfort during the infusion, that the infusion was monitored appropriately (at least once per hour), and that there were no problems during the infusion. An $800,000 verdict was awarded to the plaintiff. Intravenous Product.

S. Sinclair vs Rush-Presbyterian-St. Luke's Hosp I V line extravasation disfigures hand— $800,000 Illinois verdict. Med Malpractice Verdicts, Settlements & Experts 16(6):21–22 (Jun) 2000

INTRAVENOUS FLUIDS
Phlebitis

Over a three month period, local complications were assessed in 363 patients receiving infusion therapy after venous catheterization. The majority of cases utilized 20 gauge catheters (92%). Phlebitis occurred in 35% of the patients, usually occurring within the first few days of therapy (2.7 to 3.5 days). Risk was highest in those patients receiving antibiotics and increased as the number of antibiotics administered increased. The risk was lowest in those receiving intravenous corticosteroids.

The authors suggested that the prophylactic use of heparin and controlling drug dilution and infusion rates may be helpful in avoiding phlebitis reactions.

Intravenous Fluids
Pose-Reino A et al (Santiago, Spain) Infusion phlebitis in patients in a general internal medicine service. Chest 117(6):1822 (Jun) 2000

SEDATION (PROCEDURAL)
Overdose, Death, Legal Action

A two-year-old boy admitted for a CT scan to investigate a minor head injury associated with a fall stopped breathing after the test was completed. Results from the test indicated that there were no significant injuries. Respiratory arrest was suggested as a result of sedative overdose, administered for the procedure. Despite revival in the emergency room, the patient suffered irreversible brain damage and died five days later. A $3 million settlement was reached.

Fernandez M vs Rush-Presbyterian-St. Luke's Med Center and K Stokes. $3 million Illinois settlement reached in death of toddler after CT scan—too much sedative for scan alleged. Med Malpractice Verdicts, Settlements & Experts 16(5):26 (May) 2000

DRUGS
ALENDRONATE vs RISEDRONATE
Esophageal and Gastric Effects

In a randomized single blind multicenter study, 515 postmenopausal women were randomized to receive oral risedronate (5 mg daily) or alendronate (10 mg daily) for two weeks. At the end of two weeks, the overall incidence of gastric ulcers was significantly higher in the alendronate group (13.2% vs 4.1%). Most gastric ulcers were located in the antrum. Esophageal ulcers occurred in three and none of the alendronate and risedronate groups, respectively. Duodenal ulcers occurred in two and one of the patient groups, respectively. Overall treatment related adverse events occurred in 35.8% of the alendronate group and in 33.3% of the risedronate group. The majority of reactions were mild in both groups (69% vs 63%). The most frequently cited reactions in both groups included headache, abdominal pain, and dyspnea.

The authors concluded that alendronate was associated with a higher incidence of gastric ulcers compared to risedronate when both drugs were dosed in osteoporosis ranges. Mechanism of bisphosphonate induced gastric effects may be related to the disruption of the protectant phospholipid barrier of the gastric mucosa via displacement of phosphatidylcholine.

Lanza FL et al (Houston Instit Clin Research, 7777 Southwest Freeway, Suite 720, Houston TX 77074; e-mail:dr.lanza@pdq.net) Endoscopic comparison of esophageal and gastroduodenal effects of risedronate and alendronate in postmenopausal women. Gastroenterology 119:631–638 (Sep) 2000

ALENDRONATE
Unmasked Hypoparathyroidism

A 68-year-old woman developed dyspnea, voice hoarseness, palpitations and spasms of the larynx, hands, and tongue, approximately 10 days after starting alendronate (5 mg daily), elemental calcium (1500 mg daily), and vitamin D (800 IU daily) for osteoporosis. Other chronic medications included levothyroxine (150 mcg daily). Other symptoms included circumoral tingling and anxiety. Abnormal laboratory values indicated hypocalcemia (0.8 mmol/L), hyperphosphatemia (2.0 mmol/L) with normal thyroid hormone levels. Parathyroid hormone concentrations were decreased (14 pg/mL) for the corresponding calcium levels. Treatment included intravenous calcium chloride infusion and discontinuation of alendronate. The patient was eventually discharged on calcium carbonate (3 grams daily) and calcitriol (0.75 mcg daily). No recurrences of hypocalcemia occurred during a follow-up period of four months.

The authors concluded that alendronate induced symptomatic hypocalcemia in this patient, who was unable to compensate with increased production of parathyroid hormone because of a pre-existing unrecognized hypoparathyroidism. Thus, alendronate unmasked a subclinical case of hypoparathyroidism.

Kashyap AS & Kashyap S (Armed Forces Med Coll, Pune 411 040, India: Dept Med; e-mail:skashyap@pn2.vsnl.net.in) Hypoparathyroidism unmasked by alendronate. Postgrad Med J 76:417–419 (Jul) 2000

ALENDRONATE
Hepatotoxicity

A 71-year-old patient developed elevated liver enzyme concentrations within two months after starting alendronate (10 mg daily) for severe osteoporosis. Other chronic medications included ursodeoxycholic acid (dosage not provided). Initial elevated values included aspartate aminotransferase (118 U/L), alanine aminotransferase (163 U/L), gammaglutamyl transferase (118 U/L), and alkaline phosphatase (151 U/L). Laboratory screenings for infectious etiologies were negative but liver biopsy revealed lobular inflammation, and portal infiltration of lymphocytes, granulocytes, and eosinophils. Evidence of biliary cirrhosis was negative. Elevated liver function tests gradually normalized over a four-month period after alendronate was discontinued.

The authors concluded that liver dysfunction in this patient was related to alendronate based on the temporal relationship between drug administration and symptom development. The authors proposed possible inhibition of cholesterol synthesis as a mechanism of action. A published response from the manufacturer suggested that this event was not drug related but recurrence of previous liver dysfunction (four years earlier). Clinicians should be aware of this potential drug related event.

Halabe A et al (Edith Wolfson Med Center, 58100 Holon, Israel) Liver damage due to alendronate. N Engl J Med 343(5):365–366 (Aug 3) 2000 (letter) Daifotis AG & Yates AJ (Merck & Co, Rahway, NJ 07065) Liver damage due to alendronate. N Engl J Med 343(5):366 (Aug 3) 2000 (letter)

ALLERGY IMMUNOTHERAPY
Fatal Anaphylactic Shock, Legal Action

A 46-year-old asthmatic patient developed an allergic reaction in the physician's office after receiving a weekly allergy immunotherapy injection with newly added substance for cat dander. Treatment included diphenhydramine and epinephrine injections in the office. Approximately two months later the patient required medical treatment in the emergency room after another allergy injection. One week later, the patient developed another allergic reaction despite premedication with parenteral diphenhydramine. Additional treatment with injectable epinephrine and oxygen in the office was not enough to sustain the patient prior to the arrival of emergency medical technicians. The plaintiff claimed that the physician practiced without sufficient experience, training or monitoring of patients. Defense arguments would have included the patient's past history of asthma and allergies, and adequate management of previous allergic responses to immunotherapy. A $440,000 settlement was reached prior to trial.

Anon vs Anon. Physician's inexperience, lack of training, and failure to recognize the risk of anaphylactic shock blamed for death of woman—$440,000 Massachusetts settlement. Med Malpractice Verdicts, Settlements & Experts 16(7):3 (Jul) 2000

ALLOPURINOL
Familial Hypersensitivity

A 57-year-old man developed a generalized rash approximately two months after allopurinol (100 mg daily) and colchicine (500 mcg twice daily) were started for the treatment of gout. Previous medications included lisinopril, and a nonsteroidal anti-inflammatory agent (dosages not provided). Although the patient did not have a past history of hypersensitivity to other drugs, the patient's older brother had developed a hypersensitivity rash related to allopurinol treatment for gout. However, both patients were able to tolerate allopurinol therapy without further event after completing a desensitization regimen.

The authors concluded that a family history of allopurinol hypersensitivity may be a risk factor for other family members. It is important to note however, that both patients were able to successfully continue allopurinol therapy after completing a desensitization schedule.

Melsom RD (St. Luke's Hosp, Little Horton Lane, Bradford BD5 ONA, UK) Familial hypersensitivity to allopurinol with subsequent desensitization. Rheumatology 38:1301 (Dec) 1999 (letter)

ANESTHESIA
Reversible Sensorineural Hearing Loss

A 29-year-old patient complained of sudden deafness in the right ear and tinnitus immediately after post-operative recovery for a non-otological surgery (varicose veins). General anesthesia included induction with intravenous propofol, droperidol, fentanyl and atropine. Anesthesia was maintained with nitrous oxide and isoflurane and postoperative pain was managed with diclofenac suppository and local bupivacaine. Examination of the internal and external ear were unremarkable. However, a pure tone audiogram revealed profound sensorineural hearing loss in the right ear. Laboratory values were within normal limits and magnetic resonance imaging of the posterior cranial fossa did not indicate an acoustic neuroma. The patient was hospitalized and received treatment with regular carbogen inhalation (hourly for the first 24 hrs), intravenous Dextran 70 infusion (one liter every 12 hours for four days), oral flucloxacillin (250 mg four times daily), and oral prednisolone (60 mg daily then tapered over 11 days). Symptoms reversed to baseline after five days. The patient was discharged and audiograms performed at six weeks were within normal limits.

The authors noted that acute sensorineural hearing loss can occur after either otolaryngological and non-otolaryngological surgery. Nitrous oxide has also been implicated in previous reports.

Pau H et al. (Countess of Chester Hosp, Health Park, Liverpool Rd, Chester CH2 1UL, UK; e-mail: hpau@globalnet.co.uk) Reversible sensorineural hearing loss after non-otological surgery under general anesthesia. Postgrad Med J 76:304–306 (May) 2000

BALSALAZIDE
Allergy (First Report*)

A 59-year-old patient with intermediate patchy pancolitis was hospitalized with pain, dyspnea and back pain eight days after starting balsalazide (2.25 grams three times daily). Previous therapy included sulphasalazine. The patient was unable to tolerate mesalazine or olsalazine. Further examination revealed splinter hemorrhages beneath two fingernails and increased laboratory values, including erythrocyte sedimentation rate (122 mm/hr), C-reactive protein (251 mg/L), alkaline phosphatase (472 IU/L), gamma-glutamyl transferase (295 IU/L), alanine aminotransferase (50 U/L), and bilirubin (15 umol/L). Screenings for autoantibodies were negative but cardiac exams revealed results consistent with pericarditis and pericardial effusions. Discontinuation of balsalazide and treatment with NSAIDs resulted in symptom improvement. Pericarditis required further treatment with oral prednisolone. However, all symptoms and abnormal laboratory testing returned to baseline within a month.

The authors noted that this was the first report of allergy related to balsalazide therapy. Because the patient was able to tolerate sulphasalazine the authors suggested that the patient reacted to the balsalazide and not the sulphapyridine moiety.

Adhiyaman A et al (Withybush Gen Hosp, Haverfordwest, Pembrokeshire SA61 2PZ) Hypersensitivity reaction to balsalazide. Br Med J 320:613 (Mar 4) 2000 (letter)

COCAINE
Acute Hepatitis in HIV Patients

Three cases of acute cytologic hepatitis in HIV infected patients with nonactive viral hepatitis were documented after intranasal cocaine usage:

Patient 1: A 35-year-old HIV patient presented with acute increases in liver function tests without signs of liver dysfunction within a few days after intranasal cocaine usage. Increases in laboratory values included alanine aminotransferase (1205 IU/L), aspartate aminotransferase (851 IU/L), gamma-glutamyltransferase (196 IU/L), and alkaline phosphatase (138 IU/L). Additional elevations included CD4 count (622 cells/mm^3) and viral load (5600 RNA copies/ ml). The patient was also seropositive for Hepatitis B surface antigens. Liver biopsy was not performed. Within a few days, however, symptoms of hepatitis improved.

Patient 2: A 39-year-old HIV patient presented with hepatomegaly, fever, stiffness and sweating within a few days after intranasal cocaine usage. Increases in laboratory values included alanine aminotransferase (617 IU/L), aspartate aminotransferase (340 IU/L), gamma-glutamyltransferase (270 IU/L), and alkaline phosphatase (324 IU/L). Additional elevations included CD4 count (1236 cells/mm^3). The patient was also seropositive for Hepatitis C. Liver biopsy was not performed. Within a few days, however, symptoms of hepatitis improved.

Patient 3: A 22-year-old HIV patient presented with hepatomegaly, fever, stiffness and sweating within a few days after intranasal cocaine usage. Increases in laboratory values included alanine aminotransferase (1007 IU/L), aspartate aminotransferase (1669 IU/L), gamma-glutamyltransferase (133 IU/L), and alkaline phosphatase (519 IU/L). Additional elevations included CD4 count (1102 cells/mm^3). The patient was also seropositive for Hepatitis C. Liver biopsy was not performed. Within a few days, however, symptoms of hepatitis improved.

The authors concluded that rapid increases and decreases in liver function tests suggested that the acute hepatitis reaction in these HIV patients was related to intranasal cocaine usage. Although all patients had nonactive chronic viral hepatitis, the authors noted that viral hepatic testing remained unchanged during the acute hepatitis episode. The authors also noted that these are the first reports of hepatitis in HIV patients related to intranasal cocaine use.

Peyriere H et al (St. Charles Hosp, 34295 Montpellier, France) Cocaine induced acute cytologic hepatitis in HIV infected patients with nonactive viral hepatitis. Ann Intern Med 132(12):1010–1011 (Jun 20) 2000

COCAINE
Ischemic Colitis

Three cases of cocaine associated ischemic colitis are described.

Patient 1: A 26-year-old patient developed bloody diarrhea, cramping abdominal pain, and nausea within eight hours after smoking cocaine and marijuana. No other concurrent legal or illegal medications had been consumed, but the patient was a chronic smoker and drinker. A physical examination was unremarkable with the exception of abdominal tenderness and bright red rectal bleeding. Laboratory values included a white blood cell count (12,200/mm^3) with 69% neutrophils, hemoglobin (15 g/dL), and hematocrit (49%). Other values, including liver enzymes, were within normal ranges. A sigmoidscopy revealed a normal rectal and proximal descending colon. However, abnormalities noted in the left colon included patchy mucosal edema, erythema, and sporadic areas of submucosal hemorrhaging. Biopsy results were indicative of ischemic colitis. Treatment was not specified. Symptoms gradually improved over a 48 hour period and the patient was discharged after three days of hospitalization without further event.

Patient 2: A 41-year-old patient developed severe abdominal cramping, nausea, vomiting and bloody diarrhea during recent crack cocaine use. Medication use included hydrochlorothiazide for hypertension. A physical examination revealed abdominal tenderness without distention and bloody stools. Laboratory values included a total white blood cell count (10,100/mm^3) with 43% neutrophils and hemoglobin (15.9 g/dL). Other laboratory values were within normal ranges. A scan of the abdomen area demonstrated mucosal thickening of the sigmoid colon. Although the rectum and proximal colon were normal, biopsies demonstrated acute inflammatory cells and submucosal hemorrhages indicative of ischemic colitis. Screening for infectious etiologies was negative.

Patient 3: A 43-year-old patient was hospitalized for loss of consciousness after smoking crack cocaine and drinking alcohol for several days prior to admission. A physical examination revealed a distended and tender abdomen with hyperactive bowel sounds. Laboratory values included a total white blood cell count (18,000/mm^3) with 78% neutrophils and hemoglobin (15.9 g/dL). Other abnormal laboratory values included elevated creatinine (4.3 mg/dL), aspartate aminotransferase (78 IU/L), alanine aminotransferase (56 IU/L), lactate dehydrogenase (236 IU/L), creatine kinase (78 mg/dL), and a lactate level of 2.5 mg/dL. A sigmoidscopy revealed edematous, erythematous tissue with submucosal hemorrhages, indicative of diffuse colitis. Biopsy results confirmed ischemic colitis. During hospitalization the patient developed organ failure and bacterial sepsis eventually resulting in death within two weeks after admission.

The authors concluded that these cases of colonic ischemia were associated with cocaine usage. A suggested mechanism of action was intestinal ischemia caused by cocaine induced vasoconstriction via stimulation of the alpha-adrenergic receptors in the mesenteric arteries. It is possible that cocaine may also have a direct toxic effect on the gastrointestinal mucosa.

Linder JD et al (Monkemuller KE, Div Gastroenterol & Hepatology, 633 ZRB, UAB Station, Birmingham, AL 35294) Cocaine associated ischemic colitis. S Med J 93(9): 909–913 (Sep) 2000

CYCLOSPORINE AND ST. JOHN'S WORT
Interaction: Heart Transplant Rejection

Two cases of failed heart transplants are presented in patients who had reduced cyclosporine levels while taking the alternative medicine, St. John's Wort.

Patient #1: A 61-year-old patient previously stabilized after a heart transplant 11 months earlier was hospitalized with fatigue three weeks after starting St. John's wort (300 mg three times daily) for depression. Other chronic medications included cyclosporine (125 mg twice daily), azathioprine (100 mg daily), and corticosteroids (7.5 mg daily). Prior to St. John's wort therapy cyclosporine levels had been consistently within therapeutic range but upon admission they were decreased (95 mcg/L). Endomyocardial biopsy revealed acute cellular transplant rejection. Despite stopping St. John's wort therapy, increasing cyclosporine dosages (150 mg twice daily) and intravenous steroid dosing (1 gram/day), rejection status was unchanged. However, permanent rejection was avoided by treatment substitution with mycophenolate mofetil (1 gram twice daily) and short term intravenous anti-thymocyte globulin (1250 mg daily for 10 days). Cyclosporine levels returned to baseline levels after St. John's wort therapy was stopped.

Patient #2: A 63-year-old patient previously stabilized after a heart transplant 20 months earlier was hospitalized for elective endomyocardial biopsy three weeks after starting St. John's wort (300 mg three times daily) for anxiety and depression. Other chronic medications included cyclosporine (125 mg twice daily), azathioprine (125 mg daily), and corticosteroids (7.5 mg daily). Prior to St. John's wort therapy cyclosporine levels had been consistently within therapeutic range but upon admission they were decreased (87 mcg/L). Endomyocardial biopsy revealed acute cellular transplant rejection. Cyclosporine levels returned to therapeutic range after St. John's wort therapy was stopped and no further rejection episodes occurred during follow-up.

The authors concluded that in both patients, St. John's wort therapy was associated with a reduction in cyclosporine plasma concentrations and subsequent transplant rejection episodes. After stopping St. John's wort treatment, cyclosporine concentrations returned to therapeutic range, and rejection episodes were reversed. The authors suggested that cyclosporine levels were decreased via cytochrome P450 induction via St. John's wort. As this is an interaction with serious consequences clinicians are encouraged to avoid this combination.

Ruschitzka F et al [Division of Cardiology, Dept Internal Med, Univ Hosp, C4-8091 Zurich, Switzerland) Acute heart transplant rejection due to Saint John's wort. Lancet 355:548 (Feb 12) 2000 (letter)

CYCLOSPORIN A
Cutaneous Leucocytoclastic Vasculitis (First Report*)

A 37-year-old patient developed a purpuritic eruption on both legs approximately one month after starting cyclosporin A for psoriasis (50 mg daily). Concurrent chronic medication included indomethacin (150 mg daily). Previous unsuccessful therapies for psoriasis included oral gold (3 mg three times daily) and salazopyrine (3 grams daily). A one year course of oral cyclosporin A with another product (NeoOral) was discontinued due to side effects. Physical examination after the dermal reaction revealed necrotic ulcerations on both legs and skin biopsy showed a leucocytoclastic vasculitis with heavy dermal infiltrates. Within two months after cyclosporin A was discontinued, the eruption resolved with residual scarring. At a nine month follow-up there were no signs of vasculitis and the patient remained recurrence-free.

The authors suggested that the base ingredients of cyclosporin A were responsible for cutaneous leucocytoclastic vasculitis in this patient. They also noted that this occurred with one brand product but not with previous cyclosporin therapy with a different brand product. This suggested that the reaction was most likely due to the base products in the Sandimmun product rather than the active drug. Sandimmun contains corn oil and polyoxyethylated glycolysed glycerides as the base.

Gupta MN et al (Dept Dermatol, Monklands Hosp, Monklands Ave, Airdrie, Lanarkshire ML6 OJS) Cutaneous leucocytoclastic vasculitis caused by cyclosporin A (Sandimmun). Ann Rheum Dis 59:319 (Apr) 2000

DOPAMINE AGONISTS
Sleep Attacks

Three cases of unexpected sleep episodes are described in patients taking dopamine agonists as Parkinson's therapy, including bromocriptine, lisuride, pergolide or piribedil.

Patient 1: A 72-year-old Parkinson's patient was in an auto accident as a result of falling asleep while driving. Sleep onset was sudden and unexpected. Chronic medications included levodopa (800 mg daily) and bromocriptine (30 mg daily) for 12 and seven years, respectively. Upon further interview the patient admitted to sleepiness episodes only at rest during the previous two years. His spouse indicated that episodes were more frequent. Management of the patient and follow-up results were not provided.

Patient 2: A 55-year-old Parkinson's patient developed excessive daytime somnolence, which interfered with daily activities. Chronic medications included lisuride (1.5 mg daily), levodopa (600 mg daily), and deprenyl (10 mg daily). Somnolence improved after lisuride was discontinued. Substitution with pergolide (2 mg daily) was uneventful until the dosage was increased to 3 mg daily. Daytime sleepiness was most evident after lunch and during driving. Sleep episodes continued at an increased dosage of 4 mg daily. The patient no longer drives during pergolide therapy and holds dosages when driving is necessary.

Patient 3: A 69-year-old Parkinson's patient experienced sudden sleep episodes during the day while on levodopa (250 mg daily) and piribedil (150 mg daily) therapy. Other medications included atenolol (100 mg daily) for hypertension and diacerheine (100 mg daily) for osteoarthritis. During treatment with parkinsonism agents, the patient had an auto accident as a result of falling asleep while driving. Upon interview the patient denied daytime sleepiness, but indicated the need for a nap post lunch. Management of the patient and follow-up results were not provided.

The authors concluded that these three Parkinson's patients experienced sleep episodes most likely related to dopamine agonist therapy. Levodopa was also considered as a causative agent in one patient due to past published reports describing sedative effects. Although an exact mechanism of action was not provided, the authors suggested that this may be a drug class effect.

Ferrerira JJ et al. (Rascol O, Serv Pharmacologie, Medicale et Clinique, Faculte de Medecine, 31073 Toulouse Cedex, France; email:rascol@cict.fr) Sleep attacks and parkinson's disease treatment. Lancet 355:1333–1334 (Apr 15) 2000 (letter)

ETANERCEPT
Local Injection Site Reactions

A 51-year-old rheumatoid arthritis patient developed a large raised cutaneous reaction on the injection site of her fourth etanercept dose (dosage not provided). Other concurrent medications were not provided. The area was erythematous, warm, indurated and raised. A skin biopsy revealed superficial, perivascular infiltrates with lymphocytes and eosinophils. The drug was continued with only minor local injection site reactions.

The authors noted that local injection site reactions with etanercept are usually mild, occur one to two days after injection and last less than five days. The authors concluded that this patient experienced a mild transient inflammatory reaction that did not interfere with treatment.

Murphy FT et al (Brooke Army Med Center, 3851 Roger Brooke Dr, San Antonio, TX 78234) Etanercept associated injection site reactions. Arch Dermatol 136:556–557 (Apr) 2000 (letter)

FENFLURAMINE, PHENTERMINE
Valvular Heart Disease

The prevalence of valvular heart disease (VHD) was assessed in a prospective study of 226 obese adult outpatients receiving a phentermine-fenfluramine (phen-fen) regimen (mean age and body mass index: 46.9 yrs and 110 kg). All patients underwent transthoracic echocardiography within a mean of 97 days after the withdrawal of fenfluramine from the U.S. market. Initial doses were 15 mg/20 mg and were titrated up to 30 mg/60 mg of phentermine and fenfluramine, respectively. All subjects had a normal ECG at baseline. Concurrent medications in-cluded psychotropic and cardiac drugs in 58 of the patients and SSRIs in 20. Approximately 24 and 69 of the patients had some degree of aortic or mitral valve regurgitation, respectively. However, most cases were trace or mild in nature (18 vs 5 and 58 vs 10). Tricuspid valve regurgitation was observed in 62 and pulmonic regurgitation in 21. Significant VHD was found in 18 patients (7.9), aortic regurgitation in 15 patients and mitral disease in three patients. VHD in most patients involved only a single valve. No differences in VHD incidence was found when the data was stratified by patient age, dose, percentage weight loss, blood pressure, or mean heart rate. In addition, there was no increased prevalence of VHD in patients taking SSRIs when compared to those with disease and not taking these medications. Adverse events that occurred during the prospective study included dry mouth (87), feeling different (83), somnolence (61), sleep disturbances (60), headache (59) and confusion (51).

The authors concluded that the combination of phentermine and fenfluramine was associated with a low prevalence of significant VHD in obese patients during a prospective study. Although the exact mechanism of action has not been clearly established, previous studies have noted valvular changes consistent with patients who have ergot alkaloid induced and carcinoid valve disease.

Burger AJ et al (Div Cardiol, Beth Israel Deaconess Med Center, West Campus, Harvard Med Sch, Boston MA) Low prevalence of valvular heart disease in 226 phentermine-fenfluramine protocol subjects prospectively followed up to 30 months. J Am Coll Cardiol 34:1153–1158 (Oct) 1999

ICODEXTRIN
Allergic Reactions

A review of 102 peritoneal dialysis patients who had received icodextrin was compared to a control group of 120 continuous ambulatory peritoneal dialysis patients who received conventional glucose based dialysis over a one year period at the same dialysis center. A total of five skin reactions occurred in the icodextrin group and none in the control group. Of the reported skin reactions in the icodextrin group, three were exfoliative and two were blistering reactions on sun exposed areas. The exfoliative reactions were acute reactions which occurred soon after the first exposure (days 1 to 4) and were characterized by itching and rapidly progressing symptoms. Fever or eosinophilia was not observed. All symptoms improved within 48 hrs after icodextrin was discontinued and reversed within three weeks.

In contrast, the onset of the blistering reactions was delayed, occurring at three and six months after the initiation of icodextrin dialysis, with both occurring in the summer (July). Symptom resolution occurred over a six to eight week period. Skin biopsy revealed nonspecific inflammatory changes. None of the patients experiencing allergic episodes with icodextrin were rechallenged.

Two other cases of photosensitive skin reactions occurred with one in each group. However, both of these reactions were attributed to other causes (i.e., chronic hepatic porphyria and furosemide). Surveys of additional patients on icodextrin revealed that nine additional patients experienced skin problems, including dryness, rash and blistering.

The authors concluded that up to 15% of patients on icodextrin may experience skin reactions with symptom resolution upon withdrawal.

Goldsmith D et al (Dept Renal Med & Transplantation, 4th Floor, Thomas Guy House, Guy's Hosp, London, SE1 9RT, UK; e-mail:David.goldsmith@gstt.sthames.nhs.uk) Allergic reactions to the polymeric glucose based peritoneal dialysis fluid icodextrin in patients with renal failure. Lancet 355:897 (Mar 11) 2000 (letter)

LICORICE
Hypertension

A 38-year-old patient was hospitalized with headaches, decreased appetite, pitting edema, and hypertension (230/130 mmHg). The only medication taken was an oral contraceptive. Most laboratory values were within normal ranges with the exception of serum potassium (3.9 mmol/L), reduced urinary sodium excretion (17 mmol/L), elevated urinary cortisol (196 nmol/24 hr), decreased urinary aldosterone (1.3 nmol/24 hr), and decreased plasma renin activity (0.15 ng/L). A repeat medication history revealed the chronic ingestion of large amounts of licorice candy containing glycyrrhicinic acid (200 mg) and sodium (1.5 grams/100 grams) and licorice lozenges containing glycyrrhicinic acid (200 mg) and sodium (60 mg/100 grams). Treatment included a licorice free diet with initial therapy of urapidil followed by metoprolol, ramipril and hydrochlorothiazide. The patient initially became hypotensive which resolved when the ramipril and hydrochlorothiazide were discontinued.

The authors suggested that this patient developed hypertension as a result of the ingestion of large amounts of glycyrrhicinic acid containing licorice. Glycyrrhicinic acid is a potent inhibitor of 11-beta-hydroxysteroid dehydrogenase, an enzyme that oxidizes cortisol into cortisone. Large amounts may suppress the renin-aldosterone axis and increase urinary excretion of cortisol.

Woywodt A et al (Dept Nephrology, Univ Hannover Sch Med, Carl-Neuberg-Strasse-1, 30625 Hannover, Germany; e-mail:woywodt@aol.com) Turkish pepper (extra hot) Postgrad Med J 76:426–428 (Jul) 2000

MAGNESIUM SULFATE
Medication Error, Legal Action

An 18-year-old mother received intravenous pitocin and magnesium sulfate via separate lines through a double IMED pump during a hospitalization for delivery of her second child. Pitocin was re-ordered post placental removal, but the line delivering magnesium sulfate was inadvertently opened. Within 10 minutes the patient began thrashing then became unresponsive, requiring a resuscitation code and the administration of calcium gluconate to reverse magnesium effects. Although successfully resuscitated, the patient sustained anoxic brain damage and seizures, resulting in a vegetative state and ultimately requiring nursing home care. Liability was denied by the nurse manager and physician but admitted by the hospital. An approximate $7.4 million verdict was awarded against the hospital.

Yolanda Conley, disabled vs Advocate Health & Hosp Corp. Woman overdosed on magnesium sulfate following delivery of child—physician ordered additional pitocin, but wrong iv opened—brain damage necessitates nursing home care—$7.4 million Illinois verdict against hospital. Med Malpractice, Verdicts, Settlements & Experts 15(11):18 (Nov) 1999

ORLISTAT
Hypertension

A 40-year-old patient developed dizziness, peripheral edema, headaches, and hypertension (190/100 mmHg) after intermittent orlistat use. These symptoms developed within one week after increasing the dosage (120 mg three times daily). The patient was not taking other medications at the time. Within a few days of discontinuing orlistat, blood pressure decreased to 160/90 mmHg and further decreased to 145/95 mmHg after oral furosemide therapy (30 mg daily) was initiated. Similar symptoms recurred when orlistat was restarted two months later. Blood pressure increased to 170/100 mmHg but decreased to 140/90 mmHg after the drug was stopped. At follow-up three months later, diuretic therapy was stopped and blood pressure had stabilized at 130/90 mmHg.

The authors concluded that orlistat was responsible for hypertension in this patient based on the appearance and resolution of symptoms in relation to drug exposure. Although the exact mechanism of action was not clarified, fluid retention was suggested as a possible cause.

Persson M et al (Reg Centre for Pharmacovigilance, Karolinska Univ Hosp, SE-171 76, Stockholm, Sweden) Orlistat associated with hypertension. Br Med J 321:387 (Jul 8) 2000 (letter)

PERGOLIDE
Sleep Attacks

Two Parkinson patients who developed sleep attacks during pergolide therapy are described.

Patient 1: A 61-year-old Parkinson's patient developed increased somnolence and sleep attacks approximately one month after starting pergolide therapy (5 mg daily). Other concurrent medications included selegiline and aspirin (dosages not provided). Sleep attacks were invasive into daily functioning and occurred during talking, eating, drinking and other activities. Sleep duration ranged from several minutes to hours without further neurological complications. Sleep symptoms reversed with pergolide dosage reduction (3 mg daily).

Patient 2: A 57-year-old Parkinson's patient developed increased incidence of sleep attacks within a few weeks after being titrated to 4.5 mg of pergolide daily. There were no other medications. Sleep attacks occurred during daily activities and were unexpected. However, sleep episodes ceased after the pergolide dosage was decreased (3 mg daily).

The authors noted that sleep episodes may occur with several dopamine agonists and may be a drug class effect. They noted that the episodes associated with pergolide were sudden and unexpected and may be dangerous if they occur during driving.

Schapira AHV (Univ Dept Clin Neurosciences, Royal Free & Univ Coll Med Sch & Instit Neurology, London NW3 2PF, UK; email:schapira@rfhsm.ac.uk) Sleep attacks (sleep episodes with pergolide). Lancet 355:1332–1333 (Apr 15) 2000 (letter)

PRAMIPEXOLE
Peripheral Edema

A retrospective review of 300 patients taking pramipexole for parkinsonism or restless legs syndrome revealed that 17 developed peripheral edema during therapy. The mean age of these patients was 63.8 yrs (range: 44 to 82 yrs) with a mean onset of peripheral edema after pramipexole initiation of 2.6 months (range: 0.25 to 11 months). The mean dose at onset of the event was 1.7 mg daily (range: 0.75 mg to 3 mg daily). Peripheral edema was restricted to the ankles in 41% of the patients, at the calves in 29%, and at or above the knees in the remaining 29%. The majority of patients had difficulty walking (76%) or wearing their shoes (94%). Resolution of symptoms after drug withdrawal occurred in 16 patients. When rechallenged at lower doses, 10 of 11 patients reported similar but lessened peripheral edema symptoms within one week after restarting the medication. Two case reports were also described from this group of patients.

Patient 1: A 66-year-old parkinson's patient developed ankle edema within one week after adding pramipexole to her current regimen. Other medications included levodopa/carbidopa and amantadine. Despite symptoms, the drug was continued (titrated up to 3 mg daily) and the peripheral edema worsened, extending to above the knees. Treatment with leg elevation and furosemide resulted in only mild improvements and amantadine withdrawal did not change the course of events. However, within one week after tapering off pramipexole, the patient reported an 80% improvement in edema. Peripheral edema recurred, but to a lesser degree, within two weeks after pramipexole was started at a lower dose (0.75 mg daily). The patient was continued on the drug at this dosage.

Patient 2: A 60-year-old parkinson's patient developed bilateral ankle swelling within three weeks after pramipexole was started (1.5 mg daily). Other concurrent medications included levodopa and selegiline (no dosages provided). After titration up to 3 mg daily, edema worsened to above the knees and limiting mobility. Diuretics resulted in only mild improvement. The patient continued pramipexole (3 mg daily) with persistent edema. However, within three days after the drug was completely tapered, edema completely reversed. After reinitiation of the drug at a lower dose (1.5 mg daily), edema was restricted to the ankles.

The authors concluded that peripheral edema in these patients was a result of pramipexole therapy. They suggested that the severity of the complication was dose related. They did not identify any predisposing factors from the retrospective review. They also suggested that pramipexole induced edema is an idiosyncratic reaction.

Tan EK & Ondo W (Parkinson's Disease Center & Movement Disorders Clin Dept Neurol, Baylor Coll Med, 6550 Fannin, Smith 1801, Houston, TX 77030-3408; e-mail: wondo@bcm.tmc.edu) Clinical characteristics of pramipexole induced peripheral edema. Arch Neurol 57:729–732 (May) 2000

PROPOFOL
Green Urine

A 55-year-old inpatient developed dark green urine within three days after an intravenous propofol infusion was started for sedation during intubation. The induction dose was 40 mg (0.5 mg/kg) with a maintenance infusion of 240 mg/hr (3 mg/kg/hr). Concurrent medications included intravenous famotidine, amlodipine, fosinopril, albuterol, and ipratropium (no dosages specified). Despite the suspicion of an infectious etiology, screenings for an infectious process were negative, including urinalysis, blood cultures, and urine cultures. In addition, the white blood cell count was within normal limits and the patient remained afebrile. The urine had a dark green hue with a pH of 8.5. Within six hours of propofol discontinuation, the urine returned to baseline hue and no further sequelae ensued.

The authors concluded that propofol infusion was responsible for this patient's dark green urine, a rare but benign side effect. Possible causes for urine discoloration may include the presence of phenolic propofol metabolites in the urine, possibly promoted by an alkaline environment.

Blakely SA et al. (VA Med Center (Atlanta), 1670 Clairmont Rd, Dept 119, Decatur, GA 30033) Clinical significance of rare and benign side effects: propofol and green urine. Pharmacotherapy 20(9):1120–1122 (Sep) 2000

PROPOFOL
Violent Coughing

Six of 214 consecutive adult patients who received 1% propofol (2 mg/kg) infusions as anesthesia induction for various surgical procedures experienced violent coughing immediately after administration of the drug, lasting greater than five seconds. Five of the six patients were smokers, smoking greater than 10 cigarettes daily. Concurrent medications in all patients included oral diazepam (5 mg) on the night prior to surgery and one hour preoperatively, and intravenous glycopyrrolate (0.1 mg) prior to anesthesia induction. Opioids were not administered to any of the six patients. Violent coughing resolved after a brief period of treatment with manual ventilation (100% oxygen). Oxygen hemoglobin saturation did not decline lower than 95%.

The authors noted that these are the first case reports of propofol induced coughing. A suggested mechanism of action included airway smooth muscle contraction in response to propofol induced apnea, causing stimulation of irritant receptors. Based on these reports, the authors also questioned the use of propofol as the induction agent of choice in smokers or other patients with hyperreactive airways. They also suggested the study of prophylactic premedicants to avoid this potential complication.

Mitra S et al (Government Med Coll, Chandigarh 160047, India) Propofol induced violent coughing. Anesthesia 55:695–696 (Jul) 2000 (letter)

QUININE
Hemolytic Uremic Syndrome

A 70-year-old patient developed nausea, vomiting, mild diarrhea, bruising, and fever approximately five days after starting quinine for the treatment of nocturnal leg cramps. She ingested the first dose five days previous to the onset of symptoms, and the second dose (325 mg) six hours prior to symptom onset. Concurrent medications were not mentioned. A physical examination upon hospital admission revealed extensive bruising on the trunk and lower extremities. Abnormal laboratory values included white blood cell count ($16.2 \times 10^3/mm^3$), platelets ($37 \times 10^3/mm^3$), sodium (127 mEq/L), creatinine (9.1 mg/dL), blood urea nitrogen (100 mg/dL), and lactate dehydrogenase (8.335 U/L). Urinalysis indicated the presence of blood, protein and hyaline casts. A Coombs test and screenings for infectious etiologies were negative. Hemolytic uremic syndrome was diagnosed. Treatment included a total of 16 plasmapheresis sessions over a 37 day period and eight hemodialysis treatments during the first 23 days. Despite initial response in platelet counts, plasmapheresis was required on an outpatient basis. The patient eventually recovered without further sequelae.

The authors concluded that quinine use was responsible for hemolytic uremic syndrome in this patient and most likely developed as a result of quinine dependent antibodies to blood cellular components. It should also be noted that the FDA rescinded the approval of quinine for nocturnal leg cramps in 1995, based on lack of efficacy. Because there are no effective alternatives available, some clinicians continue to use this product for nocturnal leg cramps.

Crum NF & Gable P (Naval Med Center, Dept Internal Med, Code CCA, 34800 Bob Wilson Dr, San Diego, CA 92134-5000) Quinine induced hemolytic uremic syndrome. S Med J 93(7):726–728 (Jul) 2000

RILUZOLE
Overdose: Methemoglobinemia (First Report*)

A 43-year-old patient with amyotrophic lateral sclerosis (ALS) developed methemoglobinemia after an intentional overdose of riluzole (2.8 grams). Upon hospitalization six hours after the ingestion, the whole blood methemoglobin concentration was 18.3%. Ingestion of other medications was ruled out via a negative serum drug screening. Clinical symptoms included peripheral cyanosis and drowsiness. Laboratory measurements included arterial blood pH (7.38), a partial pressure of arterial carbon dioxide (47 mmHg), a partial pressure oxygen (73 mmHg), and oxygen saturation (95%). Treatment included gastric lavage, activated charcoal (50 grams), and intravenous methylene blue (50 mg). Mechanical ventilation was required on hospital day three for alveolar hypoventilation. Attempts to wean the patient off the ventilator were unsuccessful. The patient died on hospital day seven due to respiratory failure related to ALS.

The authors concluded that methemoglobinemia in this patient was caused by riluzole ingestion. They speculated that the drug or one of its metabolites might possess antioxidant activity, thus inducing methemoglobinemia. The manufacturers of riluzole (Aventis) also published a response following this publication, indicating that this is the first report of this type, and that the product information has been revised to reflect this new information.

Viallon A et al (Hopital Bellevue, 42055 Saint Etienne CEDEX 2, France) Shipley JE & Kugener V (Aventis Pharmaceutical Products, Bridgewater, NJ 08807-0800) Methemoglobinemia due to riluzole. N Engl J Med 343(9):665–666 (Aug 31) 2000 (letter)

RIVASTIGMINE, DONEZEPIL
Pisa Syndrome

Two cases of Pisa syndrome were reported in patients taking cholinesterase inhibitors (donezepil, rivastigmine) for Alzheimer's disease. Pisa syndrome is characterized by an abnormal leaning posture involving both the head and trunk.

Patient 1: A 53-year-old Alzheimer's patient began leaning backward and to the left approximately four weeks after starting combination therapy with risperidone (0.5 mg daily) and donezepil (5 mg daily). No other medications were mentioned. Symptoms worsened when the patient was walking. Within seven days of full withdrawal of the two drugs, symptoms resolved. Rivastigmine was initiated 10 weeks later at a dose of 3 mg, which was gradually increased to 9 mg. After seven weeks, similar dystonic symptoms and leaning were observed. However, all symptoms reversed within seven days after drug withdrawal.

Patient 2: A 73-year-old Alzheimer's patient developed left axial deviation after 16 weeks of donezepil therapy (5 mg daily). Previous therapy included risperidone (0.5 mg daily) for eight weeks. Within four weeks after donezepil was discontinued, symptoms reversed without treatment. Rivastigmine (3 mg daily) was initiated eight weeks later with symptom recurrence after only 10 days of therapy. Symptoms resolved once again within three weeks after rivastigmine was stopped.

The authors concluded Pisa syndrome developed in both patients as a result of treatment with cholinesterase inhibitors, rivastigmine and donezepil. Cholinergic excess was noted as a possible factor in the development of Pisa syndrome.

Kwak YT et al (Dept Neurology, Yong-In Hyoja Geriatric Hosp, Yongin-shi Kuseong-myeon, Sanghari 33, Kyeongki—do, 449–910, Republic of Korea; e-mail: ytkwak@netsgo.com) Relation between cholinesterase inhibitor and Pisa syndrome. Lancet 355:2222 (Jun 24) 2000 (letter) (Apr 18) 2000 (letter)

ROPINIROLE
Sleep Attacks

A 63-year-old Parkinson's patient gradually developed excessive daytime sleepiness with sleep attacks after his ropinirole daily dose was increased from 6 mg to 9 mg. Episodes of unplanned sleep occurred at least five times daily after the dosage increase. Prior treatment included low dose levodopa, which was discontinued due to mild sedation and gastrointestinal side effects. Sleep attacks reversed immediately after pergolide (1.5 mg daily) was substituted for ropinirole and symptoms remained well controlled.

The authors noted that although sedation appears to be a class effect of dopaminergic drugs, threshold doses for sedation may be different for different agents. Thus, they recommended switching to another dopamine agonist in patients with excessive sleepiness reactions.

Pirker W & Happe S (Dept Clin Neurol, Univ Vienna, A-1090 Vienna, Austria; e-mail: walter. pirker@univie.ac.at) Sleep attacks in parkinson's disease. Lancet 356:597–598 (Aug 12) 2000 (letter)

ROPINIROLE, PRAMIPEXOLE
Sleep Attacks

Two case reports of sleep attacks are described in Parkinson patients during therapy with non-ergot dopamine agonists.

Patient 1: A 66-year-old Parkinson patient experienced excessive daytime sleepiness and episodes of sleep paralysis after switching from pergolide (0.25 mg three times daily) to pramipexole (1 mg four times daily). Other chronic medications included selegiline (5 mg twice daily), benztropine (2 mg four times daily), indapamide (1.25 mg daily), and atenolol (25 mg daily). Although the pramipexole dose was slowly increased to 1 mg four times daily, the patient reported sleep episodes within two weeks after starting therapy. The episodes persisted throughout continued therapy. Treatment with modafinil (200 mg daily) was unsuccessful. Ropinirole (0.5 mg three times daily) was substituted for pramipexole therapy and slowly tapered to 1 mg three times daily. However, within one month's time the sleep episodes recurred and continued despite dosage reduction (0.75 mg three times daily). Sleep attacks did not recur after substitution with levodopa/carbidopa.

Patient 2: A 55-year-old Parkinson patient fell asleep while driving approximately one month after ropinirole (2 mg to 4 mg three times daily) was substituted for pramipexole therapy. Other medications included tolcapone (100 mg three times daily) and levodopa/carbidopa. Buspirone was prescribed for anxiety (5 mg three times daily). Additional sleep attacks occurred while driving. At this time the ropinirole dosage was 8 mg three times daily. Ropinirole was tapered and discontinued and pergolide restarted. No further sleep attacks occurred after ropinirole was discontinued.

The authors concluded that sudden sleep episodes in these patients were related to non-ergot dopamine agonist therapy. They also noted that the manufacturer of pramipexole notified health care professionals in September 1999 of this potentially dangerous side effect. The authors suggested that this adverse event may be a class effect of non-ergot dopamine agonists and that health professionals should counsel patients appropriately. An exact mechanism of action is unknown but may be related to activation of D3 receptors at lower concentrations.

Ryan M et al (Univ Kentucky Med Center, 800 Rose St C117, Lexington, KY 40536-0084) Non-ergot dopamine agonist induced sleep attacks. Pharmacotherapy 20(6): 724–726 (Jun) 2000

SILDENAFIL
Optic Neuropathy

A 52-year-old patient developed sweating, headache and blurry vision with "blue bolts" within one hour after taking one dose of sildenafil (50 mg). The only concurrent medication was methylphenidate (no dosage provided) for attention deficit disorder. Most symptoms were transient (lasting 30 minutes), but blurry vision persisted in the left eye. Rechallenge 24 hours later with another dose resulted in similar symptoms. An ophthalmic examination five days after sildenafil administration revealed an inferior altitudinal visual depression in the left eye and superior swelling of the left optic nerve head, indicating ischemic optic neuropathy.

The authors proposed that the close temporal relationship between the administration of the drug and appearance of symptoms suggested a drug induced effect. A possible mechanism of action was not provided.

Egan R et al (Casey Eye Instit, 3375 SW Terwilliger Blvd, Portland OR 97201; e-mail:eganr@OHSU.edu) Sildenafil associated anterior ischemic optic neuropathy. Arch Ophthalmol 118:291–292 (Feb) 2000 (letter)

SILDENAFIL
Priapism in Sickle Cell Trait Patient (First Report*)

A 39-year-old patient developed sustained and painful erection lasting approximately six hours after one dose of sildenafil (50 mg). Erectile dysfunction gradually worsened with complete loss of erection within three months. Physical examination was unremarkable but laboratory results were consistent with sickle cell trait.

The authors noted that priapism is a complication of sickle cell anemia but not with sickle cell trait and this report represents the first published case of sildenafil associated priapism in such a patient.

Kassim AA et al (Div Hematology, Dept Med, Albert Einstein Coll Med/Montefiore Med Center, Bronx, NY) Acute priapism associated with the use of sildenafil in a patient with sickle cell trait. Blood 95(5):1878–1879 (Mar) 2000

SIROLIMUS
Interstitial Pneumonitis

Three cases of drug induced interstitial pneumonitis were reported in renal transplant patients receiving sirolimus as immunosuppressive therapy. The ages of the patients and dosages of the drug were not provided. However, trough blood concentrations ranged from 15 to 30 ng/mL. Concurrent medications included prednisolone, aziathioprine, aspirin, acebutolol, isradipine, and gemfibrozil in Patient 1; mycophenolate, prednisolone, enalapril, furosemide, and insulin in Patient 2; and prednisolone, fenofibrate, and insulin in Patient 3. Chest x-rays and tomographic scans in all patients revealed bilateral pulmonary infiltrates. In two patients, lung function tests were restricted and exertional dyspnea gradually worsened. However, the third patient was asymptomatic. Bronchoalveolar lavage revealed lymphocytic pneumonitis in two patients, which was accompanied by intraalveolar hemorrhage in the third patient. No evidence of infectious etiology was found and none of the patients received antibiotics. After sirolimus withdrawal, clinical and radiological improvements were observed within a few weeks and interstitial pneumonitis reversed within three months.

The authors concluded that diffuse interstitial pneumonitis in these three patients was related to sirolimus therapy based on the temporal relationship between drug administration and the appearance and resolution of symptoms. A mechanism of action was not provided. The authors also suggested that this reaction might be misdiagnosed as an infectious process in transplant patients on immunosuppressive therapy. Thus, clinicians should consider this potential reaction in patients taking sirolimus who present with pneumonitis.

Morelon E et al. (Hosp Necker, 75743 Paris CEDEX 15, France) Interstitial pneumonitis associated with sirolimus therapy in renal transplant recipients. N Engl J Med 343(3):225 (Jul 20) 2000 (letter)

SODIUM POLYSTERENE SULFATE-SORBITOL
Colonic Necrosis

A 61-year-old inpatient developed abdominal pain 24 hours after the first dose of sodium polysterene-sorbitol enema (SPS-45 grams). Another dose was administered orally (30 grams). Other medications administered prior to this dose included insulin (20 units), calcium gluconate (two ampules), and glucose (two ampules). Symptoms progressed to hypothermia, tachycardia, and hypotension requiring phenylephrine. Because of an acute abdominal tenderness and distention, the patient underwent an emergency laparotomy, which revealed a mottled transverse colon. However, the remainder of the colon and abdominal content were normal. Examination of the removed transverse colon revealed necrotic mucosa. The post-operative course was uneventful and the patient was discharged to a rehabilitation facility within three weeks.

The authors concluded that SPS-sorbitol was responsible for colonic necrosis in this patient. Renal dysfunction may have been a co-factor. Although an exact mechanism of action is not known, possible suggestions included hypovolemia, hyperreninemia, elevated prostaglandin production, and localized mesenteric vasospasm. In addition, improper administration of SPS-sorbitol was also provided as a possible but unlikely cause. The authors cautioned all prescribers to be aware of this possible serious complication associated with either the oral or rectal administration of SPS-sorbitol.

Dardik A et al. (Harrison MC, Sinai Hosp of Baltimore, 2435 Belvedere Ave, Suite 42, Baltimore, MD 21215) Acute abdomen with colonic necrosis induced by kayexalate sorbitol. S Med J 93(5):511–513 (May) 2000

SUMATRIPTAN
Mesenteric Ischemia

Two cases of mesenteric ischemia are described in two adult patients.

Patient 1: A 45-year-old patient developed abdominal cramping, bloody diarrhea and hypotension within hours after administering a subcutaneous injection of sumatriptan (up to ten 6 mg doses per week). A total of four episodes occurred with one episode requiring hospitalization for right hemicolectomy for transmural necrosis. After stopping sumatriptan therapy, the patient was without side effects during a 14-month follow-up period. However, two similar episodes occurred after 14 months while not on sumatriptan therapy.

Patient 2: A 63-year-old patient developed abdominal pain and bloody diarrhea within hours after taking oral sumatriptan (50 mg) for migraine therapy. A flexible sigmoidoscopy revealed ischemic colitis. Symptoms did not recur during a four month follow-up period after sumatriptan withdrawal.

The authors concluded that mesenteric ischemia was related to sumatriptan in these patients. Although an exact mechanism of action was not provided, the authors noted that this drug has potent vasocontrictive activities. They cautioned clinicians to consider mesenteric ischemia in patients taking sumatriptan who develop abdominal pain or hematochezia.

Liu JJ (Mayo Clin & Foundation, Rochester MN 55905) Sumatriptan associated mesenteric ischemia. Ann Intern Med 132(7):597 (Apr 4) 2000 (letter)

TACROLIMUS
Autoimmune Diabetes

A 32-year-old diabetic developed antibodies for glutamic acid decarboxylase (GAD: 55.1 U/mL) with worsening glycemic control (19.7 mmol/L) within five months after a liver transplant. Medications included tacrolimus (10 mg daily) and azathioprine (50 mg daily). In addition, glucagon stimulated serum C-peptide level indicated pancreatic B-cell dysfunction (0.1 nmol/L). Despite reversal of GAD antibody status, pancreatic B-cell dysfunction persisted.

The authors suggested that tacrolimus may cause a "chemical diabetes" via pancreatic beta cell injury or by binding to receptors for adenosine diphosphate ribose in pancreatic beta cells.

Kawai T et al (Keio Univ Sch Med, Tokyo, Japan 160-8582) FK 506-induced autoimmune diabetes. Ann Intern Med 132(6):511 (Mar 21) 2000 (letter)

TEMOPORFIN
Light Exposure Burns

A total of 14 healthy adult men were enrolled in a pharmacokinetic study in which they received a single dose of temoporfin (0.1 to 0.129 mg/kg). Sunlight exposure after two weeks produced a photosensitivity reaction in two men. The remaining individuals were instructed to avoid prolonged sunlight exposure over the next three months. Within 48 hours after discharge from the study, six of the 12 men developed partial thickness burns on the left forearm and other burns after short term sun exposure. Treatment at regional burn centers included paraffin dressings. Prolonged recovery was observed with scarring in some individuals.

The authors suggested that these photosensitive reactions were related to temoporfin therapy.

Hettiaratchy S & Clark J. (Regional Burns Centre, Chelsea & Westminister Hosp, London SW109NH) Burns after photodynamic therapy. Br Med J 320:1245 (May 6) 2000

THALIDOMIDE
Toxic Epidermal Necrolysis

A 64-year-old patient with myeloma developed a rash 10 days after a thalidomide dosage increase. Initial therapy included thalidomide 200 mg daily for two weeks followed by 400 mg daily. Concurrent therapy included dexamethasone. Within three days after rash onset, symptoms progressed to erythema on the trunk, face and extremities accompanied by blistering and oral and oropharynx ulcerations. Skin biopsy confirmed full thickness epidermal necrosis. The patient recovered after two weeks.

The authors cautioned regarding a possible drug interaction between thalidomide and dexamethasone, increasing the risk of serious skin reactions. They recommended that this combination not be used until additional information is collected. They also suggested that thalidomide not be used with other drugs known to cause serious skin reactions (e.g. sulfonamides, allopurinol).

Rajkumar SV et al. (Mayo Clinic, Rochester MN 55905) Life-threatening toxic epidermal necrolysis with thalidomide therapy for myeloma. N Engl J Med 343:972 (Sep 28) 2000

THALIDOMIDE
Toxic Epidermal Necrolysis (First Report*)

A 62-year-old woman developed a full-body maculopapular rash approximately five weeks after starting thalidomide (titrated up to 600 mg daily) for glioblastoma. She had a history of previous allergic responses manifested as rash when exposed to phenytoin and erythromycin on separate occasions. Other concurrent medications during this event included phenobarbital. The rash slowly resolved over the next five days after both thalidomide and phenobarbital were discontinued and divalproex was started. However, the patient visited the emergency room when she developed a flare of the rash, dyspnea and pruritus, approximately eight hours after receiving a rechallenge dose of oral thalidomide (100 mg). Other symptoms upon admission included hypotension (80/40 mmHg), tachycardia (100 beats/min), and dyspnea (20 breaths/min). The rash covered her entire body with bullous lesions primarily on the shoulders and chest. Superficial sloughing was also noted on the back. Other concurrent medications upon admission included oral dexamethasone (8 mg daily), divalproex (250 mg four times daily), nizatadine (150 mg twice daily), diphenhydramine (25 mg four times daily) and bisoprolol (50 mg daily). Initial treatment included intravenous dexamethasone (10 mg), diphenhydramine (50 mg), famotidine (20 mg) for a suspected allergic reaction and potassium chloride (30 mEq) for hypokalemia. Other medications also included gentamicin (200 mg daily), vancomycin (1 gram daily) and analgesics (propoxyphene-acetaminophen). During hospitalization the rash worsened involving significant desquamation and transfer to a burn unit for three weeks before discharge.

The authors noted that this was the first published case of thalidomide induced toxic epidermal necrolysis. Although phenobarbital was recognized as a possible factor, the authors suggested rashes occur much earlier during phenobarbital treatment courses. The authors cautioned clinicians to be aware of this potentially serious reaction and to implement treatment as early as possible when recognized.

Horowitz SB et al (A. Stirling, St. John's Univ Coll Pharmacy & Allied Health Prof, 8000 Utopia Pkway, Jamaica, NY 11439) Thalidomide induced toxic epidermal necrolysis. Pharmacotherapy 19(10): 1177–1180 (Oct) 1999

TRASTUZUMAB
Serious Adverse Events, FDA Notification

On May 3, 2000, the FDA and manufacturer of trastuzumab notified health professionals regarding 62 postmarketing reports of serious adverse events associated with the use of this drug. Serious events included hypersensitivity reactions, infusion and pulmonary reactions. Fifteen of these reactions were fatal and nine developed symptoms within 24 hours after infusion. Based on these postmarketing reports the product labeling was changed to include a boxed warning which specified hypersensitivity reactions including fatal anaphylaxis, potentially fatal infusion reactions, and pulmonary reactions (including adult respiratory distress syndrome and death). In most patients, symptoms began with the first dose of trastuzumab, usually within 12 to 24 hours. In patients with fatal reactions, most had pre-existing pulmonary dysfunction. If one of these reactions occur therapy should be discontinued immediately.

Serious adverse events with trastuzumab.(www. fda.gov/medwatch/safety/2000/hercep. htm) (May 3) 2000

ZUCLOPENTHIXOL
Neutropenia, Thrombocytopenia (First Report*)

A 66-year-old patient was hospitalized with thrombocytopenia and neutropenia approximately 18 days after zuclopenthixol (10 mg three times daily) was added to his regimen. Other medications included glyburide (5 mg three times daily), biperiden (2 mg twice daily), oxazepam (10 mg three times daily), dipyridamole (75 mg three times daily), and ranitidine (150 mg once daily). Although reductions in both leukocytes (2.9×10^9 cells/L) and platelets ($10^9 \times 10^9$/L) upon admission, there was no evidence of clinical bleeding. Within five days after zuclopenthixol was discontinued, the white blood cell and platelet count increased (3.7×10^9 cells/L and 134×10^9/L, respectively). Follow-up post discharge revealed values within normal limits.

The authors concluded that zuclopenthixol was responsible for this patient's hematological abnormalities. A mechanism of action was not provided.

Hirschberg B et al (Caraco Y, Div Internal Med, Clin Pharmacol Unit, Hadassah Univ Hosp, PO Box 12000, Jerusalem 91120, Israel; e-mail:caraco@hadassah.org.il) Zuclopenthixol associated neutropenia and thrombocytopenia. Ann Pharmacother 34: 740–742 (Jun) 2000

RESPIRATORY AGENTS
RESPIRATORY AGENTS
RESPIRATORY AGENTS
RESPIRATORY AGENTS
RESPIRATORY AGENTS
RESPIRATORY AGENTS

Drug	ADR	Page Number
Beclomethasone	Growth velocity reduction	217
Beta-agonists (inhaled)	Myocardial infarction risk	218
Fluticasone	Pulmonary aspergillosis	218
Ipratropium (Nebulized)	Dilated pupils	219
Ipratropium (Inhaled)	Blurred vision	219
Montelukast	Churg-Strauss syndrome	220
Theophylline	Seizures in epileptic children	220
Zafirlukast	Hepatic dysfunction	221

Respiratory Agents

BECLOMETHASONE, FLUTICASONE (Inhaled)
Growth Velocity Reduction

A total of 159 trials of inhaled steroid therapy were identified for inclusion in a meta-analysis to determine the effects of inhaled therapy on linear growth in children. Of these, only five trials met the criteria for the meta-analysis, including a randomized controlled trial which included children with asthma in the study and providing greater than 12 weeks of inhaled steroid therapy. Four of the five trials used inhaled beclomethasone (328 to 400 mcg daily) and one study used inhaled fluticasone (200 mcg daily). Analysis of the four beclomethasone trials demonstrated a significant reduction in linear growth in children with mild to moderate asthma who received inhaled beclomethasone when compared to children with a nonsteroid medication (−1.51 cm/year). In the fluticasone study, there was a mean difference of −0.43 cm/year between 96 children treated with inhaled fluticasone and 87 treated with placebo.

The authors concluded that moderate doses of inhaled beclomethasone or fluticasone may decrease growth velocity in children with asthma. However, the authors also noted that these conclusions are based on only one fluticasone study, and that the magnitude of effect with fluticasone was smaller than that of beclomethasone. In addition, the effects, if any, on final adult height are not known.

Sharek PJ & Bergman DA (Lucile Packard Children's Hosp at Stanford, 725 Welch Rd, Palo Alto, CA 94304; e-mail:psharek@leland.stanford.edu) The effect of inhaled steroids on the linear growth of children with asthma: A meta-analysis. Pediatrics 106(1):1–7 (Jul) 2000 http://www.pediatrics.org/cgi/content/ full/106/1/e8

217

BETA-AGONISTS (Inhaled)
Myocardial Infarction Risk

The risk and incident myocardial infarction was assessed in a case control study enrolling 1,444 cases and 4,094 controls. Cases included patients who experienced an incident fatal or nonfatal myocardial infarction over a 5.5 year period. Both cases and controls were assessed for metered dose inhaler (MDI) use of beta-agonists and defined as never users, one-time users and regular users. For all subjects, the adjusted odds ratio (OR) was 1.67 for subjects who received one MDI canister compared to those who did not receive an MDI beta agonist during the three month period previous to their myocardial event. The OR was also elevated for those subjects who received two to four MDI canisters in the three months prior to the index date. However, in patients with a history of cardiovascular disease and who had used one MDI canister in the three month period, the OR was significantly higher (3.22). In contrast, those without cardiovascular disease were without increased risk (0.89). Use of two or more canisters in the previous three months was not associated with an increased risk of myocardial infarction regardless of the presence of cardiovascular disease. When subset use was examined, the estimated risk of myocardial infarction was highest among new users who had used a canister within three months previous to the event (7.32). Frequent (greater than one-time) users who had filled prescriptions for more than one MDI beta-agonist within the previous three months had an estimated risk of 1.78.

The authors concluded that new users of inhaled beta-agonists with cardiovascular disease may be at increased risk of myocardial infarction. They also cautioned clinicians to consider this information when prescribing new inhaled beta-agonist therapy in patients with cardiovascular disease.

Au DH et al (Div Pulmonary & Crit Care Med, Harborview Med Center, Univ Washington, Box 359762, 325 Ninth Ave, Seattle, WA 98104-2499) The risk of myocardial infarction associated with inhaled beta-adrenoreceptor agonists. Am Respir Crit Care Med 161:827–830 (Mar) 2000

FLUTICASONE (Inhaled)
Invasive Pulmonary Aspergillosis (First Report*)

A 44-year-old patient developed pulmonary aspergillosis during inhaled fluticasone therapy (440 mcg four times daily) for moderately severe asthma. Other concurrent medications included oral zafirlukast (20 mg daily). Hemoptysis also developed. Initial treatment with oral itraconazole was unsuccessful, warranting therapy with an investigational antifungal medication (nonspecified). A chest x-ray revealed bilateral cavitary lesions, which was confirmed as chronic necrotizing aspergillosis after an open lung biopsy. A cosyntropin stimulation test during therapy indicated adrenal insufficiency and the dosage of inhaled fluticasone was tapered. Repeated scans noted improvement in pulmonary lesions and clinical symptoms abated after the drug was tapered.

The authors noted that fluticasone is the most potent inhaled steroid available in the United States and was most likely responsible for the development of systemic effects in this patient who had no known history of immunosuppression. They also noted that this is the first report of invasive pulmonary aspergillosis associated with an inhaled corticosteroid. They cautioned clinicians to be aware of these potential risks when prescribing highly potent corticosteroid formulations.

Leav BA et al (New England Medical Center, Boston, MA) Invasive pulmonary aspergillosis associated with high-dose inhaled fluticasone. N Engl J Med 343(8):586 (Aug 24) 2000 (letter)

IPRATROPIUM BROMIDE (Inhaled)
Blurred Vision

A 68-year-old patient with chronic obstructive pulmonary disease complained of blurred vision for seven years. Chronic medications during that time included ipratropium bromide oral inhalation (two puffs every six hours), orally inhaled albuterol, aspirin, bisacodyl, calcium carbonate, diltiazem, fluticasone propionate nasal spray, ibuprofen, lisinopril, lorazepam, salmeterol, sucralfate, multivitamin, and prednisone. An eye exam revealed vision of 20/100. When repeated two days later after ipratropium was held, vision had improved to 20/40.

The authors concluded that vision problems in this patient were related to ipratropium therapy. No mechanism of action was provided. They cautioned clinicians to consider this possibility in patients with vision changes who are taking ipratropium.

Kizer KM et al. (VA Med Center, Pharmacy Dept, 1310 24th Ave South, Nashville, TN 37212-2637; e-mail:Bess.david_t@nashville.va.gov) Blurred vision from ipratropium bromide inhalation. Am J Health Syst Pharm 57:996 (May 15) 2000 (letter)

IPRATROPIUM BROMIDE (Nebulized)
Unilateral Fixed Dilated Pupil

An 11-month-old inpatient developed a unilateral fixed dilated pupil shortly after completing a course of inhalation therapy on the fourth day with nebulized ipratropium bromide (0.5 mL, 250 mcg/mL) and salbutamol (0.25 mL, 5 mg/mL). Clinical and neurological examination did not indicate alternative etiologies. The dilated pupil lasted approximately 18 hours with spontaneous resolution.

The authors concluded that possible temporary incorrect positioning of the face mask may have occurred during aerosol inhalation, causing topical exposure to one eye in this patient. They cautioned that clinicians should be aware of this potential reaction and that care should be taken to position the face mask appropriately to avoid this type of reaction.

Woelfe J et al (Children's Hosp, Univ Bonn, Bonn, D-53113, Germany) Unilateral fixed dilated pupil in an infant after inhalation of nebulized ipratropium bromide. J Pediatrics 136(3):423 (Mar) 2000 (letter)

MONTELUKAST
Churg-Strauss Syndrome

A 72-year-old asthmatic developed coughing, dyspnea, ankle edema, polyarthralgia and digit paraesthesias approximately 10 days after starting montelukast (10 mg daily). Concurrent therapy included inhaled fluticasone (750 mcg twice daily) and inhaled salmeterol (50 mcg twice daily) but oral corticosteroids had not been taken for at least three months. Symptoms continued to progress and a physical examination after one month of montelukast therapy revealed wheezing and inspiratory crackles with decreased respiratory peak flow (290 L/min) and reduced FEV/FVC (1.23/1.46 mL/min). Upon hospitalization, a rash and fever were also discovered. Abnormal laboratory values included C-reactive protein (28.7×10^9/L), rheumatoid factor (282 IU/mL), eosinophils (54.7%), and albumin (30 g/L). Chest x-rays also revealed bilateral basal infiltration. Screenings for infectious etiologies were negative. Montelukast and salmeterol therapy were discontinued. Treatment included oral prednisolone (30 mg daily), analgesics, and azathioprine (1 mg/kg daily). Pulmonary symptoms and rash resolved quickly, but the peripheral neuropathy persisted. Hematological parameters returned to baseline values.

The authors noted that this is the first report of Churg-Strauss Syndrome in a patient taking montelukast therapy in the absence of oral corticosteroid withdrawal. They concluded that montelukast was responsible for this reaction based on the temporal relationship between the drug and adverse effects, and previous reports in the literature between other leukotriene receptor antagonists and similar reactions. They also advised that clinicians monitor for systemic symptoms in patients during leukotriene receptor antagonist therapy.

Tuggey JM & Hosker HSR (Hosker HSR, Dept Resp Med, Airedale Gen Hosp, Keighley, West Yorkshire, BD20 6TD, UK) Churg-Strauss syndrome associated with montelukast therapy. Thorax 55:805–806 (Sep) 2000

THEOPHYLLINE
Seizures in Children with Epilepsy

In a retrospective review of 143 epileptic children in an outpatient clinic, 43 had previously received theophylline. Of these children, 16 experienced seizures during theophylline therapy. Six patients were excluded because the seizures were thought to be related to factors other than theophylline. The remaining 10 patients were compared to 27 epileptic children who did not experience seizure during theophylline therapy. When the group was compared for age, gender, epilepsy type, anticonvulsants, and theophylline duration and dosage, the only factor that correlated with theophylline seizures was age. Infants under the age of one year experienced a higher incidence of theophylline seizures when compared to those older than one year. In three children with convulsions, theophylline concentrations were below 10 mcg/mL.

The authors concluded that infants less than one year are at higher risk of experiencing theophylline induced seziures and that this agent should be avoided in this age group. They suggested that the ratio of free theophylline to total serum concentration of the drug is high in neonates and may predispose this age group to toxicity.

Miura T et al (Dept Pediatrics, Haga Red Cross Hosp, Tochigi, Japan) Theophylline induced convulsions in children with epilepsy. Pediatrics 105(4):920 (Apr) 2000

ZAFIRLUKAST
Dear Health Professional Letter, Hepatic Dysfunction

On September 15, 2000, the FDA and the manufacturer of zafirlukast (AstraZeneca) notified health professionals of significant revisions in the safety section of the product labeling. Based on postmarketing surveillance data, revisions addressed more specific recommendations regarding patient management in the event of liver dysfunction. New recommendations include the discontinuation of the drug with immediate monitoring of liver function tests. If zafirlukast induced liver dysfunction is suspected, zafirlukast therapy should not be resumed. Postmarketing surveillance data also noted that most hepatic events occurred in women. Additional revisions all addressed the increased risk of adverse events, with the exception of infections, in the elderly population. Other adverse events added to product labeling include arthralgia and myalgia.

Hepatic dysfunction with zafirlukast. (Sep) 2000 http://www.fda.gov/medwatch/safety/2000/accola.htm

SKIN

SKIN

SKIN

SKIN

SKIN

SKIN

Drug	Interacting Drug	ADR	Page Number
Benzocaine		Methemglobinemia	225
Camphor (topical)		Hepatotoxicity*	226
Doxepin (topical)		Mental status alteration (child)	227
Isotretinoin		Teratogenicity	227, 228
Lidocaine		Metallic taste	230
Lidocaine (solution)		Seizures^	229
Mentholatum		Delirium*	230
Methylsalicylate	Warfarin	Anticoagulation potentiation	231
Prilocaine		Methemglobinemia	231
Salicylic acid		Amputation from sore (+)	232
Tazarotene (topical)		Pyogenic granuloma lesion*	232

* = first report
^ = death
(+) = legal action

Skin

BENZOCAINE
Methemoglobinemia

A 71-year-old inpatient with pneumonia developed central cyanosis and decreased saturated oxygen pressure (84%) shortly after bronchoscopy and endotracheal intubation. During the procedure two doses of 20% benzocaine were sprayed over one second and were separated by approximately two hours. An arterial blood gas sample revealed a pHa of 7.43, $PaCO_2$ of 40 mmHg, PaO_2 of 201 mmHg, and an arterial percent oxygen saturation gap of 9%. The methemoglobin level was 22.5% indicating methemoglobinemia. Treatment included intravenous methylene blue 1% (1 mg/kg) for five minutes with reversal within one hour. A repeated arterial blood gas sample revealed a pHa of 7.40, $PaCO_2$ of 41 mmHg, PaO_2 of 129 mmHg, SaO_2 of 99% and SpO_2 of 96%. At this time the methemoglobinemia level was 2.4%. Approximately 2.75 hours post methylene blue dose, the SaO_2 and the SpO_2 were 98%. Antimicrobial treatment for pneumonia was continued without event and no recurrences of methemoglobinemia recurred.

The authors concluded that this patient had several underlying disease factors, which contributed to CO_2 retention and hypoxemia. However, an unaffected PaO_2 and SaO_2 suggested that methemoglobinemia was caused by topical benzocaine spray. They suggested that clinicians should be aware of this potential complication which may go unrecognized in critically ill patients.

Nguyen ST et al (Bashour CA: Dept Cardiothoracic Anesthesia, Cleveland Clinic Foundation, 9500 Euclid Ave, G-5, Cleveland, OH 44195) Benzocaine induced methemoglobinemia. Anesth Analg 90:369–371 (Feb 1) 2000

BENZOCAINE/TETRACAINE/BUTYL AMINOBENZOATE
Methemoglobinemia

An 80-year-old patient developed hypoxia after undergoing a trans-esophageal echocardiography in which he received three one-second pharyngeal sprays of Cetacaine. Oxygen saturation decreased to 85% and was not reversed after the administration of 100% oxygen. Other medications included chlorpropamide (100 mg daily), furosemide (80 mg daily), enalapril (20 mg daily), sustained release metoprolol (50 mg daily), potassium chloride (20 mEq daily), warfarin (3 mg daily), sertraline (50 mg daily), tramadol (50 to 100 mg every four to six hours as needed), docusate sodium (250 mg twice daily), and insulin. The methemoglobin concentration was 40.7%. Treatment included intravenous methylene blue (80 mg) resulting in rapid return of oxygen saturation levels to 95%. Two units of packed red cells were also administered, improving the hematocrit (31.6%).

The authors concluded that this case of methemoglobinemia was associated with local anesthetic use. They also stated that rapid recognition of this potential life threatening complication is essential in initiating appropriate treatment.

Gregory PJ & Matsuda K (Natural Med Comprehensive Database, 3120 W March Lane, Stockton, CA 95208; e-mail:pgregory@pletter.com) Cetacaine spray induced methemoglobinemia after transesophageal echocardiography. Ann Pharmacotherapy 34:1077 (Sep) 2000 (letter)

CAMPHOR (Topical)
Hepatotoxicity (First Report*)

A 2-month-old patient was hospitalized for right inguinal area swelling and failure to thrive. Most laboratory values were within normal ranges, including hematological parameters, glucose levels, electrolytes, urinalysis, and thyroid and kidney function. However, by day four of hospitalization, liver function tests were markedly elevated, including alanine transferase (225 IU/L), aspartate aminotransferase (684 IU/L), alkaline phosphatase (266 IU/L), and lactate dehydrogenase (738 U/L). Clotting tests were within normal limits. An abdominal ultrasound revealed a normal liver. Although the infant was not taking any medications, the mother revealed that she applied a topical cold remedy containing camphor three times a day to the baby's chest for five days prior to the initial hospitalization. Liver function tests gradually improved with an uneventful recovery period and the child was discharged. The mother was instructed not to apply the cold medicine. Follow-up during a three month period revealed normal liver function tests and a thriving child.

The authors concluded that this case of acute hepatotoxicity was related to the generous application of topical camphor, which resulted in systemic absorption. They also noted that this is the first case report describing hepatotoxic effects after dermal application.

Uc A et al (Betton Clin, 1505 W 11th St, Little Rock, AR 72202) Camphor hepatotoxicity. S Med J 93(6):596–598 (Jun) 2000

DOXEPIN (Topical)
Altered Mental Status in Child

A five-year-old child was hospitalized for difficulty in arousal within 24 hours after an entire tube of doxepin 5% cream (30 grams) was applied topically for a pruritic rash over a 24 hour period. There were no concurrent medications. Upon admission the child was responsive only to painful stimuli; however, there were no neurological abnormalities observed and laboratory values were within normal limits. Serum concentrations of doxepin and its metabolite, desmethyl-doxepin, were 11.95 and 17.71 ng/mL, respectively. Remaining product was removed by extensive washing with soap and water. Within 18 hours the patient had fully recovered and was discharged.

The authors noted that this was only the second case report of doxepin toxicity related to a dermal exposure in a child. They also encouraged clinicians to be aware of this potential toxicity and to select appropriate products for pruritis.

Zell-Kanter M et al (Div Occupational Med, Cook County Hosp, 1900 W Polk St, Suite 500, Chicago, IL 60612) Doxepin toxicity in a child following topical administration. Ann Pharmacother 34:328–329 (Mar) 2000

ISOTRETINOIN
Pregnancy Exposure: Teratogenic Complications

Isotretinoin, a known teratogen, has been on the market for over a decade for the treatment of severe recalcitrant nodular acne. Because of recognized teratogenic effects, the manufacturer of isotretinoin has developed an extensive pregnancy prevention program to avoid isotretinoin use during pregnancy. This program has been in existence for approximately 10 years (1989 to 1999) in which time 454,273 women of reproductive age taking isotretinoin have enrolled. In March 1999, 23 California women who used isotretinoin while pregnant were identified, of which 14 consented to interviews. These women had a median age of 25.5 yrs (range: 15 to 39 yrs) and approximately half (57%) admitted to sexual intercourse during isotretinoin therapy without contraceptive protection. Almost all (93%) did not use two forms of contraception as recommended by product guidelines. Although all of the interviewees admitted that they knew isotretinoin should not be used during pregnancy, all of these women also indicated that they did see all parts of the pregnancy prevention program materials, and four only read the information available on the drug packet. In addition, none of the women were referred to free contraceptive counseling as provided by the pregnancy prevention program. The following three case reports detail results of isotretinoin exposed pregnancies.

Patient #1: A 25-year-old woman took isotretinoin for one month during an unrecognized pregnancy. Although the first pregnancy test was negative, the second one was positive and the woman did not wait for menstruation before starting isotretinoin therapy as recommended by product information. The infant was born with numerous anomalies including congenital heart disease, which was unresponsive to medical surgical treatment, resulting in death at nine weeks.

Patient #2: A 35-year-old woman took isotretinoin for approximately 12 weeks during pregnancy. She had been on chronic therapy for approximately six months. This was her third isotretinoin exposed pregnancy and the only one to result in a live birth. Although the first course of therapy was provided by a dermatologist, subsequent courses were provided by a health care worker who was known to the patient as a friend. The infant was born without event or deformities.

Patient #3: A 35-year-old woman using isotretinoin for only one week prior to menstruation for oily skin took two doses during pregnancy. She was not under medical supervision during these courses and had been using the drug in this manner for approximately three years. The medication was obtained via a health care provider who was a friend and the patient had not been counseled regarding the need for contraception. The pregnancy was terminated.

The CDC summary noted that this information does not represent all women taking isotretinoin, and cannot be extrapolated to represent all isotretinoin-exposed pregnancies. However, this information does emphasize the importance for medically supervised courses of therapy in appropriate candidates who would be compliant with stringent criteria regarding contraceptive practices during isotretinoin use.

Anon. Accutane exposed pregnancies—California 1999. Morbidity Mortality Weekly Report 29(2):28–31 (Jan 21) 2000

ISOTRETINOIN
Tetratogenicity: Temporal Bone Anomalies

An infant exposed to isotretinoin in utero during the first trimester was born with several anomalies, including but not limited to congenital hydrocephalus, mental retardation and a seizure disorder. Because of severe retardation, auditory testing was not performed although hearing deficits were suspected. After a fatal cardiac arrest at the age of 4.5 years, an autopsy revealed several additional anomalies including undescended testes, splenomegaly, CNS malformations and multiple anomalies of the external, middle and inner ear. The temporal bones of the ear were malformed including the malleus, incus and stapes. Bone marrow protrusions were found in the middle ear cavity, external auditory canals and mastoid. The patient also had a narrow external hypoplastic facial nerve, absent chorda tympani nerve and stapedius muscle.

The authors noted that although isotretinoin is a recognized teratogen, administration during an undetected pregnancy still remains a possibility despite rigorous criteria to prevent such an event. They also cautioned clinicians to be aware that ear anomalies may also occur in patients with isotretinoin syndrome resulting from in utero exposure.

Ishijima K & Sando I (Elizabeth McCullough Knowles Otopathology Lab, Div Ophthalmol, Dept Otolaryngology, Univ Pittsburgh Sch Med, Pittsburgh, PA) Multiple temporal bone anomalies in isotretinoin syndrome. Arch Otolaryngol Head Neck Surg 125:1385–1388 (Dec) 1999

LIDOCAINE (Solution)
Seizures, Death

A 21-year-old patient developed seizures and respiratory distress while gargling 4% lidocaine solution (20 mL or 800 mg) for 60 seconds for throat anesthesia in preparation for an outpatient esophageal gastroduodenoscopy. The patient was not taking other medications, was instructed not to swallow the lidocaine solution, and did not have a prior history of cardiac or respiratory disease. Other symptoms included hypotension and severe bradycardia. Despite treatment with oxygen, intubation, intravenous midazolam and hydrocortisone (500 mg), his condition worsened with subsequent death.

The authors noted that the dose used in this patient (800 mg) was greater than the recommended maximum dose (200 mg) commonly used in throat anesthesia. Rapid absorption was most likely responsible for CNS and cardiovascular toxicity. They also noted that this was the first report of death associated with lidocaine toxicity when used for esophageal gastroduodenoscopy. The authors recommended that lidocaine use for local anesthesia should be dosed at less than 200 mg and patients should be specifically instructed not to swallow the medication.

Zuberi BF et al (5 Professors' Colony, Chandka Med Coll Larkana, Pakistan; e-mail:bader@workmail.com) Lidocaine toxicity in a student undergoing upper gastrointestinal endoscopy. Gut 46:435 (Mar) 2000 (letter)

LIDOCAINE
Metallic Taste Sensation

A 73-year-old woman developed a pronounced metallic taste sensation shortly after receiving local lidocaine 2%/bupivicaine 0.375% injections prior to cataract surgery. Specifically, a Nadbath block behind the left pinnea was performed. Other chronic medications at the time of surgery included glyburide, clonidine and lovastatin (no dosages provided). Examination after the injections indicated motor blockade of the left seventh nerve and first, third and sixth cranial nerves. After a successful surgery lasting approximately 1.5 hours, the metallic sensation persisted. The patient was unable to distinguish between salt and sugar solutions placed on the anterior left side of the tongue, but had no problem identifying the solutions on the right side of her tongue. Taste sensations were normal on follow-up 24 hours later.

The authors concluded that the Nadbath block with lidocaine resulted in a sensory block of the anterior left tongue possibly caused by a blockade of the sensory branch of the seventh cranial nerve and resulting in a metallic taste by the patient.

Bigeleisen PE (Div Reg Anesthesia, Univ of Rochester Sch Med & Dentistry, Strong Mem Hosp, Rochester, NY 14642) An unusual presentation of metallic taste after lidocaine injections. Anesth Analg 89:1239–1240 (Nov) 1999

MENTHOLATUM
Delirium (First Report*)

A 63-year-old nursing home resident was hospitalized three times during a one year period for altered mental status after repeated intentional ingestion of Mentholatum. Shortly after ingestion the patient experienced euphoria, confusion, lethargy, visual and audio hallucinations, and behavioral changes. Psychiatric evaluation during the third hospital admission revealed underlying memory deficits, borderline intellectual functioning and deficits in visuospatial skills. A physical examination also revealed an edematous and fissured tongue, generalized muscular atrophy, lipid pneumonia, chronic obstructive pulmonary disease and mild hypoxemia. Confusion decreased during the hospital stay.

The authors concluded that periodic mentholatum ingestion was responsible for this patient's episodes of delirium. Underlying cognition deficits may have also contributed to the events. The authors cautioned clinicians to be aware of this potential abuse syndrome with resultant toxicities.

Huntimer CM & Bean DW (Sioux Falls, SD) Delirium after ingestion of mentholatum. Am J Psychiatry 157:483–484 (Mar) 2000

METHYL SALICYLATE (Topical) AND WARFARIN
Interaction: Anticoagulation Potentiation

A 22-year-old patient previously stabilized on warfarin therapy for one month had elevated INRs (12.2) after applying topical 7% menthol/0.05% methyl salicylate to both knees for eight nights. The patient was not taking any other medications during the previous four weeks. Dietary changes also included increased spinach consumption. Increased bruising and bleeding of the gums after brushing was also observed. Management included oral vitamin K (2.5 mg), holding the next warfarin dose, and stopping gel application. The next INR decreased to 5.0. Reinstitution of warfarin at previous dosages resulted in therapeutic INRs during follow-up monitoring.

The authors concluded that topical salicylate therapy was responsible for anticoagulation potentiation in this patient. Possible mechanisms included systemic salicylate absorption in amounts sufficient to affect vitamin K metabolism or displacement of warfarin via protein binding. Clinicians are encouraged to discuss this interaction with patients who may use topical salicylate products.

Joss JD & LeBlond RF (Dept Pharmaceutical Care, Univ Iowa Health Care, 200 Hawkins Dr, Iowa City, IA 52246; e-mail:jacqueline-joss@uiowa.edu) Potentiation of warfarin anticoagulation associated with topical methyl salicylate. Ann Pharmacother 34:729–733 (Jun) 2000

PRILOCAINE (Peribulbar Blockade)
Methemoglobinemia

A 27-year-old diabetes mellitus patient developed tachypnea, somnolence and decreased saturated oxygen pressure (87%) within 60 minutes after a peribulbar blockade was administered during retinal surgery. The peribulbar anesthesia consisted of prilocaine (80 mg), bupivacaine (30 mg), hyaluronidase (no dosage provided), and naphazoline (no dosage provided). Chronic medications included captopril (25 mg daily), verapamil (240 mg daily), isosorbide dinitrate (40 mg daily), and furosemide (40 mg daily). Although an electrocardiogram and breath sounds were normal, an arterial blood gas revealed a PaO_2 of 236 mmHg, $PaCO_2$ of 32 mmHg, a pH of 7.31 and hemoglobin level of 5.3 g/dL. The methemoglobin level was 11.2%. Improvement in blood gas values occurred shortly after intravenous methylene blue was administered (1.5 mg/kg). The remainder of the patient's surgery and hospital stay was uneventful.

The authors concluded that small amounts of prilocaine, administered as peribulbar blockade, might cause methemoglobinemia in patients who have reduced tolerance to oxidant drugs. Other factors, which may have contributed to this case, included a possible unrecognized genetic predisposition in this patient to methemoglobinemia formation and/or the chronic administration of nitrates.

Eltzschig H et al (Schroeder TH, Channing Lab, Brigham and Women's Hosp, Harvard Med Sch, 181 Longwood Ave, Boston, MA 02115) Methaemoglobinemia after peribulbar blockade: an unusual complication in ophthalmic surgery. Br J Ophthalmol 84(4):442 (Apr) 2000 (letter)

SALICYLIC ACID
Sore Resulting in Amputation, Legal Action

A 72-year-old diabetic removed a wart with prescribed salicylic acid pads that were applied on his foot for a two week period. The acidic pad caused a sore on the sole of the foot, which was resistant to healing and ultimately became infected. Despite treatment, the infection worsened due to the patient's diabetic condition and ultimately required amputation of the leg below the knee. The plaintiff claimed that the use of salicylic acid pads for diabetics was outside the standard of care. The defense experts refuted this claim. The defense also claimed that other physicians provided poor care. A reported settlement of $300,000 was reached.

Anon vs Anon Use of salicylic acid pads to remove a wart from a diabetic's foot blamed for sore which led to amputation—North Carolina settlement for $300,000. Med Malpractice Verdicts, Settlements & Experts 16 (4):52 (Apr)2000

TAZAROTENE (Topical)
Pyogenic Granuloma Lesion (First Report*)

During a controlled clinical trial of topical tazarotene (0.1%) gel for scalp psoriasis, one patient developed a pyogenic granuloma in the treated area after two weeks of therapy. No further lesions developed during continued use of the product for an additional 10 weeks. Biopsy confirmed the diagnosis.

The authors noted that pyogenic granulomas have been reported with oral retinoids but have not been associated with topical retinoid use. They suggested that there may be a relationship which requires further study. No mechanism of action was provided.

Dawkins MA et al (Dept Dermatol, Wake Forest Univ Sch Med, Medical Center Blvd, Winston-Salem, NC 27157-1071) Pyogenic granuloma like lesion associated with topical tazarotene therapy. J Am Acad Dermatol 43(1):154–155 (Jul) 2000 (letter)

VACCINES/SERUMS
VACCINES/SERUMS
VACCINES/SERUMS
VACCINES/SERUMS
VACCINES/SERUMS
VACCINES/SERUMS

Drugs	ADR	Page Number
Anthrax vaccine	Adverse events	235
Antithymocyte globulin	Acute renal failure*	236
BCG vaccine	Peritonitis*	237
BCG vaccine	Systemic granulomatous disease	236
Botulinum toxin	Extraocular muscle damage*	238
Botulinum toxin	Respiratory failure*	237
Hepatitis B vaccine	Optic neuritis	239
Hepatitis B vaccine	Neonatal ADRs	238
Immune globulin	Myocardial infarction	240
Immune globulin	Hemolytic anemia	239
Influenza vaccine	Perocarditis	241
Polio vaccine	Optic neuritis	239
* = first report		

Vaccines/Serums

ANTHRAX VACCINE
Adverse Events

In December 1997, the U.S. Department of Defense initiated the Anthrax Vaccination Immunization Program (AVIP), a phased vaccination program to protect military personnel against potential anthrax use as a biological weapon by the year 2004. As of April 20, 2000 approximately 426,000 service personnel had received an estimated 1.6 million doses of adsorbed anthrax vaccine. A survey of 6879 service members in Korea from September to October 1998 revealed that approximately 37% were receiving their first dose, and the remainder were receiving either the second or third doses. Most respondents reported localized minor reactions, which spontaneously resolved without treatment. However, women reported higher reaction rates to previous vaccine doses than men. Approximately 2% of all vaccinees reported limited work performance after vaccination, and 0.3% reported < one day loss from work after the first or second vaccination dose. In a cohort of approximately 603 service personnel receiving the vaccination in Hawaii, approximately 8% of the vaccinees reported muscle or joint aches, headache and fatigue requiring medical attention or time from work after the first dose. Similar reactions were reported by 5%, 3% and 3% after the second, third and fourth doses, respectively.

The CDC concluded that these findings suggest that rates of local reactions were higher in women than in men but there were no patterns of unexpected local or systemic reactions identified. It was noted that the method of adverse detection and reporting was subject to several limitations, including small sample size and underreporting.

CDC. Surveillance for adverse events associated with anthrax vaccination. U.S. Department of Defense 1998–2000. Morbidity and Mortality Weekly Report 49(16):341–45 (Apr 28) 2000

235

ANTITHYMOCYTE GLOBULIN
Acute Renal Failure (First Report*)

A 36-year-old inpatient developed fever and increased BUN (47 mg/dL) within 24 hours after receiving antithymocyte globulin (4.2 grams) for the treatment of aplastic anemia. Other indications of renal dysfunction included elevated laboratory parameters including, creatinine (3.4 mg/dL), urine pH (5), specific gravity (1.015) and hematuria. Other medications included cyclosporine A, which was decreased from 1.3 grams daily to 400 mg daily prior to admission for the antithymocyte globulin administration. Serum cyclosporine concentration was 231 ng/dL. No abnormalities were observed via renal ultrasound. BUN and creatinine continued to increase, peaking at 94 mg/dL and 5.2 mg/dL, respectively, on post-administration day three. By day six, these values had decreased to 35 mg/dL and 1.0 mg/dL, respectively.

The authors concluded that this was the first published report of antithymocyte induced renal failure. They also suggested that cyclosporine may have contributed to the antithymocyte induced renal injury, although an exact mechanism of action was not provided.

Levine IM & Lien YHH (Univ of Arizona Coll Med, Tucson, AZ) Antithymocyte globulin induced acute renal failure. Am J Kidney Diseases 24(6).1115 (Dec) 1999 (letter)

BACILLUS CALMETTE GUERIN VACCINE
Systemic Granulomatous Disease

A 75-year-old patient with a recent history of transitional cell carcinoma of the urinary bladder was hospitalized for chronic fever during the last two months prior to admission. The only medication was monthly intravesical instillations of bacillus calmette guerin (BCG) vaccine with the last installation performed approximately one month prior to admission. Laboratory values upon admission revealed thrombocytopenia (82 × 10^9/L) and increased liver function tests, including aspartate aminotransferase (40 U/L), gamma-glutamyltransferase (254 U/L), alkaline phosphatase (566 U/L) and pancreatic lipase (720 U/L). A chest scan also revealed an infiltration surrounding the pleural space. Biopsies of the liver and bone marrow revealed granulomas with both epitheloid and giant cells but cultures of this material were unsuccessful. Mycobacterium bovis, however, was isolated from urine specimens. Treatment with isoniazid, rifampicin and ethambutol resulted in rapid clinical recovery and laboratory values returned to baseline within one week. Treatment was discontinued five months later without symptom recurrence.

The authors concluded that the systemic disease in this patient was related to inoculation via BCG administration in the bladder. The authors also cautioned clinicians to monitor for symptoms of systemic infection in patients receiving BCG vaccine.

Mooren FC et al (Depts Med B & Pathology, Westfalische Wilheims-Univ, Munster, Germany) Systemic granulomatous disease after intravesical BCG instillation. Br Med J 320:219 (Jan 22) 2000 (letter)

BACILLUS CALMETTE GUERIN (Intravesical)
Peritonitis (First Report*)

A 69-year-old diabetic patient on peritoneal dialysis developed a chronic low grade fever and abdominal pain after three months of weekly intravesical instillations of bacillus calmette guerin (BCG) for bladder cell carcinoma. Infectious etiologies were negative and a CT scan showed nonspecific abdominal distention. Peritoneal biopsy revealed granulomatous peritonitis and fluid infected with mycobacterium tuberculosis, which responded within two weeks of isoniazid and rifampin therapy (no dosages provided).

The authors noted that this is the first case of BCG induced peritonitis and suggested that peritoneal dialysis may have increased the risk via direct inoculation or bacteria translocation. They cautioned clinicians to carefully monitor patients taking BCG while on peritoneal dialysis.

Kim IY et al (Scott Dept Urology & Div Nephrology, Baylor Coll Med, 6560 Fannin, Suite 1400, Houston, TX 77030) Bacillus calmette guerin induced peritonitis in a patient on dialysis. J Urology 163:237 (Jan) 2000 (letter)

BOTULINUM TOXIN
Botulism Like Syndrome, Respiratory Failure
(First Report*)

A 30-year-old woman was hospitalized with ptosis, catatonia, and syncope within six hours after receiving a second dose of botulinum toxin (8 × 12.5 units) in the posterior neck muscle for cervical dystonia. During hospitalization symptoms progressed to loss of gag reflex and respiratory arrest, requiring intubation and mechanical ventilation. Complete spontaneous recovery occurred within 18 hours. The authors noted that this is the first case report of respiratory failure associated with botulinum toxin injections used within therapeutic ranges. Although the drug is usually considered safe and effective, the toxin often produces local relaxation of surrounding muscles when administered. The authors cautioned clinicians about this potential life threatening adverse event possibly related to local botulinum toxin injections.

Cobb DB et al. (Univ Texas Health Science Center at San Antonio, South Texas Poison Center, 7703 Floyd Curl Dr, Mail Code 7849, San Antonio, TX 78229-3900) Botulism like syndrome after injections of botulinum toxin. Vet Human Toxicol 42(3):163 (Jun) 2000

BOTULINUM TOXIN
Permanent Extraocular Muscle Damage (First Report*)

A 70-year-old man with chronic right hyperphoria developed permanent loss of the left inferior rectus muscle function after a single local botulinum toxin A injection (2.5 units). The only other medication was phenelzine (15 mg daily). Although EMG muscle response was low to moderate post-injection, the procedure was uneventful. However, the patient complained of double vision during a one month follow-up visit, which persisted without improvement over the next 10 months. Atrophy of the left inferior rectus muscle was verified via magnetic resonance imaging. Surgery to correct this complication was successful.

The authors noted that this was the first published report of permanent damage to an extraocular muscle after botulinum toxin A injection and was possibly caused by intramuscular hematoma or direct damage. The authors cautioned clinicians to be aware of this rare complication.

Mohan M et al (Fleck BW: Princess Alexandra Eye Pavilion, Chalmers St, Edinburgh EH3 9HA) Permanent extraocular muscle damage following botulinum toxin injection. Br J Ophthalmol 83(11):1309–1310 (Nov) 1999 (letter)

HEPATITIS B VACCINE
Neonatal Events

In a retrospective review of postmarketing adverse events reported to the National Vaccine Adverse Event Reporting System (VAERS) from January 1991 to October 1998, 1771 reports were received regarding adverse effects occurring in neonates after the administration of the Hepatitis B vaccine. Of these reports, 18 resulted in death. Of the reported deaths, eight and nine occurred in boys and girls, respectively and in one report, gender was not noted. The mean age at the time of vaccination was 12 days (range: one to 27 days) with a median symptom onset of two days post vaccination (range: 0 to 20 days). Death occurred as early as the same day of symptom onset to as late as 15 days post-symptom development. In 16 cases, the causes of death, as determined by medical examiners, were most often related to sudden death syndrome (12) and infection (3).

The authors recognized that VAERS reports are voluntary and do not imply incidence nor establish a causal relationship between the hepatitis B vaccine and these events. They also noted that approximately 86 million doses of the pediatric hepatitis B vaccine have been administered since 1991 and initial data suggests that Hepatitis B vaccine may not increase the risk of neonatal death.

Niu MT et al (FDA, Center for Biologic Evaluation & Research, Div Biostats & Epidemiology, 1401 Rockville Pike, HFM-210, Rockville, MD 20852; e-mail:niu@cber.fda.gov)

Neonatal deaths after hepatitis B vaccine: the vaccine adverse event reporting system, 1991–1998. Arch Pediatr Adolesc Med 153:1279–1282 (Dec) 1999

HEPATITIS B VACCINE AND POLIO VACCINE
Bilateral Optic Neuritis

A 44-year-old woman developed gradual vision loss and retrobulbar pain upon eye movement approximately seven days after receiving vaccinations for hepatitis B and poliomyelitis. An ocular exam revealed optic nerve swelling causing decreased vision which worsened over the next 48 hours. Treatment included intravenous methylprednisolone (1 gram daily) for five days followed by oral prednisolone (1 mg/kg/day). Vision remained impaired at a three month follow-up examination. All hematological and biochemical laboratory values were within normal limits.

The authors concluded that the vaccines were most likely responsible for optic neuritis in this patient based on the appearance of symptoms post administration. An exact mechanism of action, however, was not provided. Possible causes may include immune complex mediated demyelination or neurotoxicity, or hypersensivity.

Stewart O et al (Dept Ophthalmology, Bradford Royal Infirmary, Bradford, West Yorkshire) Simultaneous administration of hepatitis B and polio vaccines associated with bilateral optic neuritis. Br J Ophthalmology 83:1200–1201 (Oct) 1999 (letter)

IMMUNE GLOBULIN (Intravenous)
Hemolytic Anemia

A 5-month-old infant with Kawaski's disease developed severe autoimmune hemolytic anemia after receiving intravenous immune globulin (400 mg/kg/day). Relevant hematological parameters included a red blood cell count of 2.55×10^6/uL and a hemoglobin of 6.8 g/dL which further decreased to 1.89×10^6/uL and 4.8 g/dL, respectively. Anti-A antibodies (1:512) and positive direct and indirect Coombs test were also documented. Treatment with intravenous prednisone (1.5 mg/kg/day) resulted in initial improvement. The remainder of the patient's hospital course included thrombi in a left coronary aneursym and an acute myocardial infarction. The authors suggested that autoimmune hemolytic anemia probably developed in this patient as a result of a high dose (4 g/kg) of immunoglobulin. No mechanism of action was provided.

Nakagawa M et al (Dept Peds, Shiga Univ Med Science, Seta, Otsu, Shiga, Japan) Severe hemolytic anemia following high dose intravenous immunoglobulin administration in a patient with Kawaski disease. Am J Hematology 63(3):160–161 (Mar) 2000

IMMUNE GLOBULIN
Acute Myocardial Infarction Associated with High Doses

Four cases of acute myocardial infarction (MI) after high dose administration of immune globulin in patients with autoimmune disorders are discussed.

Patient 1: A 60-year-old man with relapsing polychondritis refractory to prior therapy, developed severe retrosternal pain radiating to his arms three days after completing a three day regimen of intravenous immune globulin infusion (IVIG: 660 mg/kg/day infused over eight hours). An electrocardiogram revealed ST segment depression (2 mm) and abnormal labs included creatine kinase (560 u/mL), suggesting an acute MI. Although the patient's course was marked by ventricular arrhythmia and first degree AV block, recovery was eventually complete.

Patient 2: A 41-year-old woman with a history of coronary heart disease with polymyositis refractory to prior treatment developed atypical chest pain immediately after receiving the second dose of IVIG (1000 mg/kg/day infused over eight hours). However, an EKG was normal and the patient completed one year of IVIG infusions. After the last infusion she experienced exertional retrosternal pain without changes on EKG or thallium-dipyridamole heart scan. Six months later azathioprine and monthly IVIG treatments were reinitiated. Three days after the third IVIG dose, she experienced severe retrosternal pain with another normal EKG. However, three days later after another episode of severe chest pain she fainted and an EKG revealed increased ST segments. Elevated laboratory levels included serum creatine kinase, MB fraction and troponine levels. Recovery was uneventful.

Patient 3: A 67-year-old man with chronic inflammatory demyelination polyneuropathy refractory to steroids developed severe retrosternal pain within a few hours after his first dose of IVIG (400 mg/kg/day). EKG changes and increased creatine kinase levels were suggestive of an acute myocardial infarction, which required cardiac catheterization and angioplasty. Further IVIG treatment was continued (400 mg/kg/day over six to seven hours) under cardiac monitoring without event.

Patient 4: A 67-year-old man with severe immune cytopenias related to Kaposi sarcoma developed transient right hemiparesis within 24 hours after receiving two doses of IVIG (400 mg/kg/day over eight hours). A CT scan of the brain confirmed a stroke. IVIG therapy was continued and after two additional doses the patient suffered a MI. Recovery was uneventful.

The authors concluded that IVIG caused MIs in these patients and suggested that the risk of IVIG related vascular events may be higher in older patients, those who have hypertension, a history of stroke or coronary heart disease. Other reports from the literature are reviewed.

Elkayam O et al (Dept Rheumatology, Tel Aviv "Sourasky" Med Centre, 6 Weizman St, Tel Aviv, 64329, Israel) Acute MI associated with high dose intravenous immunoglobulin infusion for autoimmune disorders: A study of four cases. Ann Rheum Dis 59:77–80 (Jan) 2000

INFLUENZA VACCINATION
Pericarditis

Two cases of benign acute pericarditis were described in patients who received influenza vaccinations.

Patient 1: A 75-year-old man was hospitalized for fever, shivering, arthralgias and chest pain which developed six days after receiving an influenza vaccination. Chest pain worsened upon deep inspiration. Most laboratory values were within normal limits with the exception of white blood cell count ($16,200/mm^3$) with 92% neutrophils, C-reactive protein (13.2 mg/dL), and creatinine (2.6 mg/dL). Laboratory screenings for infectious etiologies were negative. Although a 12 lead ECG was normal, an echocardiogram revealed a small pericaridal effusion. Treatment included aspirin (1 gram three times daily), which resulted in clinical improvement within 10 days after aspirin was initiated and pericardial effusion was completely resolved upon a repeat echocardiogram at 30 days. The aspirin was discontinued after one month of therapy.

Patient 2: A 40-year-old man was hospitalized shortly after receiving an influenza vaccination. Symptoms upon admission included intermittent acute chest pain, tachycardia (100 bpm), and fever. A 12 lead ECG revealed normal sinus rhythm with PR depression and ST elevation, indicative of a myocardial infarction. However, coronary angiography and angioplasty were normal. Acute pericarditis was diagnosed after a clear pericardial friction rub was heard. The patient was discharged on aspirin therapy after three days of hospitalization.

The authors suggested that influenza vaccination with resultant subclinical influenza activity was related to the development of acute pericarditis in these patients. They noted that this diagnosis was supported by a significant increase in antibodies against influenza virus.

DeMeester A et al (Jolimont Hosp, 7100 Haine-Saint-Paul, Belgium) Symptomatic pericarditis after influenza vaccination. Report of two cases. Chest 117(6):1803–1805 (Jun) 2000

Drug Interaction Index

Drug	Interacting Drug	ADR	Page Number
Amitriptyline	Venlafaxine	Serotonin syndrome	130
Amprenavir	Ketoconazole	Increased concentrations	23
Antiretroviral	Methylprednisolone	Immunosuppression(+)	21, 175
Buspirone	Fluoxetine	Serotonin syndrome*	124
Calcium carbonate	Levothyroxine	Levothyroxine absorption reduced	156, 177
Ceftazidime	Vancomycin	Ocular precipitation (intravitreal)	33
Celecoxib	Warfarin	Coagulation changes	76, 103
Cerivastatin	Gemfibrozil	Rhabdomyolysis	89
Ciprofloxacin	Glyburide	Hypoglycemia(resistant)	40, 167
Ciprofloxacin	Warfarin	Hypothrombinemia, bleeding	41, 77
Cisapride	Grapefruit juice	Cisapride concentrations increased	157
Clarithromycin	Itraconazole	Clarithromycin concentrations increased	35
Clarithromycin	Omeprazole	Omeprazole concentrations increased	34, 159
Creatine	Ma Huang	Ischemic stroke*	8
Cyclosporine	St. John's wort	Cyclosporine concentrations decreased	10, 11, 196
Dextromethorphan	Pseudoephedrine	Psychosis	148
Digoxin	St. John's wort	Digoxin levels decreased	11, 91
Diltiazem	Simvastatin	Simvastatin concentrations increased	92
Fentanyl	Ritonavir	Fentanyl clearance decreased	27, 109
Fluorouracil	Warfarin	INR prolonged	56, 78
Fluoxetine	Buspirone	serotonin syndrome*	124
Gabapentin	Propranolol	Dystonia	95, 115

Drug	Interacting Drug	ADR	Page Number
Gemcitabine	Warfarin	INR prolonged	56, 79
Gemfibrozil	Cerivastatin	Rhabdomyolysis	89
Glyburide	Ciprofloxacin	Hypoglycemia (resistant)	40, 167
Grapefruit juice	Cisapride	Cisapride concentrations increased	157
Grapefruit juice	Methylprednisolone	Methylprednisolone concentrations increased	175
Haloperidol	Imipenem	Hypotension	136
Imipenem	Haloperidol	Hypotension	136
Indinavir	St. John's wort	indinavir concentrations decreased	9, 25
Itraconazole	Clarithromycin	Clarithromycin concentrations increased	35
Ketoconazole	Amprenavir	Increased concentrations	23
Levothyroxine	Calcium carbonate	Levothyroxine absorption reduced	156, 177
Ma Huang	Creatine	Ischemic stroke*	8
Meperidine	Ritonavir	Meperidine concentrations increased	28, 110
Methadone	Ritonavir	Methadone effect decreased	28, 111
Methylprednisolone	Antiretroviral	Immunosuppression(+)	21, 175
Methylprednisolone	Grapefruit juice	Methylprednisolone concentrations increased	175
Methylsalicylate	Warfarin	Anticoagulation potentiation	79, 231
Miconazole (vaginal)	Warfarin	INR increased	19, 80
Nabumetone	Warfarin	INR increased*	81, 107
Nefazodone	Trazodone	Serotonin syndrome*	125
Omeprazole	Clarithromycin	Omeprazole concentrations increased	34, 159
Paroxetine	Risperidone	Serotonin syndrome*	127
Propranolol	Gabapentin	Dystonia	95, 115
Pseudoephedrine	Dextromethorphan	Psychosis	148
Risperidone	Paroxetine	Serotonin syndrome	127
Ritonavir	Fentanyl	Fentanyl clearance decreased	27, 109
Ritonavir	Meperidine	Meperidine concentrations increased	28, 110
Ritonavir	Methadone	Methadone effect decreased	28, 111
Simvastatin	Diltiazem	Simvastatin concentrations increased	92
St. John's wort	Cyclosporine	Cyclosporine concentrations decreased	10, 11, 196

Drug	Interacting Drug	ADR	Page Number
St. John's wort	Digoxin	Digoxin levels decreased	11, 91
St. John's wort	Indinavir	Indinavir concentrations decreased	9, 25
Tolterodine	Warfarin	INR prolonged	81
Trazodone	Nefazodone	Serotonin syndrome*	125
Trifluoperazine	Venlafaxine	Neuroleptic malignant syndrome*	129
Vancomycin	Ceftazidime	Ocular precipitation (intravitreal)	33
Venlafaxine	Amitriptyline	Serotonin syndrome	130
Venlafaxine	Trifluoperazine	Neuroleptic malignant syndrome*	129
Warfarin	Celecoxib	Coagulation changes	76, 103
Warfarin	Ciprofloxacin	Hypothrombinemia, bleeding	41, 77
Warfarin	Fluorouracil	INR prolonged	56, 78
Warfarin	Gemcitabine	INR prolonged	56, 79
Warfarin	Methylsalicylate	Anticoagulation potentiation	79, 231
Warfarin	Miconazole (vaginal)	INR increased	19, 80
Warfarin	Nabumetone	INR increased*	81, 107
Warfarin	Tolterodine	INR prolonged	81

* = first report
(+) = legal action

FDA/Manufacturer Alert Index

Drug	Interacting Drug	ADR	Page Number
Abacavir		Hypersensitivity reactions	21
Alosetron		Ischemic colitis, constipation	155
Amprenavir		Propylene glycol toxicity (potential)	23
Aristolochic Acid		Nephrotoxicity	3
Cisapride		Cardiac toxicity	157
Cisapride		Market withdrawal due to ADRs	158
Epoetin		Pyrogenic reactions	73
Indinavir	St. John's wort	Indinavir concentrations decreased	25
Misoprostol		Pregnancy contraindication	159
St. John's wort	Indinavir	Indinavir concentrations decreased	9, 25
Streptokinase		Hypersensitivity, off-label use	75
Thioridazine		QT Prolongation	139
Trastuzumab		Serious ADRs	213
Troglitazone		Market withdrawal due to ADRs	170
Valproic acid		Pancreatitis	120
Zafirlukast		Hepatic dysfunction	221

First Report Index

Drug	Interacting Drug	ADR	Page Number
Alatrovafloxacin		Thrombocytopenia*	38
Amitriptyline		Hypersensitivity reaction*	123
Anabolic steroids		Renal cell carcinoma*	174
Balsalazide		Allergy*	193
BCG vaccine		Peritonitis*	237
Botulinum toxin		Extraocular muscle damage*	237
Botulinum toxin		Respiratory failure*	238
Brimonidine		Psychosis*	148
Buspirone	Fluoxetine	Serotonin syndrome*	124
Camphor (topical)		Hepatotoxicity*	226
Chlorambucil		Hepatic failure*	52
Chromium picolinate		Exanthematous pustulosis*	4
Ciprofloxacin		Bullous pemphigoid*	39
Clopidogrel		Hemolytic uremic syndrome*	70
Clozapine		Intersitital nephritis*	132
Creatine	Ma Huang	Ischemic stroke*	8
Cyclosporin A		Leucocytoclastic vasculitis*	197
Dalteparin		Alopecia*	72
Diltiazem		Oral ulcerations*	92
Divalproex sodium		Thermoregulatory dysfunction*	113
Doxazosin		Priapism*	94
Fluoxetine		Pheochromocytoma precipitation*	124
Fluoxetine	Buspirone	Serotonin syndrome*	124
Fluticasone		Pulmonary aspergillosis	218
Glimperide		Thrombocytopenic purpura*	167
Infliximab		Increased susceptibility: listeriosis*	158
Interferon-alpha		Diabetic ketoacidosis*	57
Interferon-beta		Focal neuropathy*	59

249

Drug	Interacting Drug	ADR	Page Number
Kampo		Epithelial keratopathy*	7
Ketoprofen		Acute renal failure*	106
Lamotrigine		Agranulocytosis*	116
Levofloxacin		QT prolongation*	42
Ma Huang	Creatine	Ischemic stroke*	8
Mentholatum		Delirium*	230
Methotrexate		Allergic reaction (first dose)*	60
Miconazole (vaginal)	Warfarin	INR increased*	19
Nabumetone	Warfarin	INR increased*	81, 107
Nefazodone	Trazodone	Serotonin syndrome*	125
Oxaliplatin		Hemolytic anemia^*	61
Paroxetine	Risperidone	Serotonin syndrome	127
Propylthiouracil		Disseminated intravascular coagulation*	178
Riluzole		Methemglobinemia (overdose)*	205
Risperidone	Paroxetine	Serotonin syndrome	127
Rofecoxib		Renal failure in transplant patient*	108
Sildenafil		Priapism in sickle cell*	208
Tazarotene (topical)		Pyogenic granuloma lesion*	232
Thalidomide		Toxic epidermal necrolysis*	212
Trazodone	Nefazodone	Serotonin syndrome*	125
Trifluoperazine	Venlafaxine	Neuroleptic malignant syndrome*	129
Trovafloxacin		Demylinating polyneuropathy*	43
Venlafaxine		Bruxism*	129
Venlafaxine	Trifluoperazine	Neuroleptic malignant syndrome*	129
Warfarin		Hemmorrhage mimics pelvic tumor*	76
Warfarin	Miconazole (vaginal)	INR increased*	19
Zuclopenthixol		Neutropenia, thrombocytopenia*	213

* = first report

Legal Action Index

Drug	Interacting Drug	ADR	Page Number
Allergy immunotherapy		Anaphylactic shock^ (+)	191
Antiretroviral	Methylprednisolone	Immunosuppression(+)	21, 175
Dobutamine		Infitration (+)	93
Fentanyl		Overdose due to heated patch^ (+)	109
Gentamicin		Neurotoxicity, ototoxicity (+)	18
Haloperidol		Medication error, overdose (+)	135
Heparin		Thrombocytopenia (+)	74, 75
Ibuprofen		Renal failure^ (+)	105
Magnesium sulfate		Medication error (+)	201
Methotrexate		Med error, overdose (+)	60
Methylprednisolone	Antiretroviral	Immunosuppression (+)	21, 175
Morphine		Self dosing pump error, resp arrest (+)	111
Prednisone		Hip necrosis, med error (+)	176
Prednisone		Osteonecrosis (+)	176
Salicylic acid		Amputation from sore (+)	232
Tetracycline		Pseudotumor cerebri (+)	47
Timolol		Respiratory arrest (+)	151
Triamcinolone		Infection, scarring (+)	177
Trimethoprim-Sulfamethoxazole		Stevens Johnson syndrome^ (+)	44

^ = death
(+) = legal action

Newly Marketed Drugs: 1997-2000

Drug	Drug Class	Year Approve	Interacting Drug	ADR	Page Number
Abacavir	Antiinfective-antiviral	1998		Hypersensitivity reactions^	21
Abacavir	Antiinfective-antiviral	1998		Hypersensitivity reactions	21
Alatrovafloxacin	Antiinfective-quinolone	1997		Thrombocytopenia*	38
Alosetron	Gastrointestinal	2000		Ischemic colitis, constipation	155
Amprenavir	Antiinfective-antiviral	1999		Propylene glycol toxicity (potential)	23
Amprenavir	Antiinfective-antiviral	1999	Ketoconazole	Increased concentrations	23
Balsalazide	Gastrointestinal	2000		Allergy*	193
Celecoxib	CNS-NSAID	1998	Warfarin	Coagulation changes	103
Celecoxib	CNS-NSAID	1998		Pancreatitis	103
Celecoxib	CNS-NSAID	1998		Auditory hallucinations	102
Celecoxib	CNS-NSAID	1998		Gastropathy, hypthrombinemia	101
Cerivastatin	Cardiac-antilipemic	1997	Gemfibrozil	Rhabdomyolysis	89
Cerivastatin	Cardiac-antilipemic	1997		Rhabdomyolysis	88
Clopidogrel	Blood	1997		Acute arthritis	69
Clopidogrel	Blood	1997		Ageusia	69
Clopidogrel	Blood	1997		Thrombotic thrombocytopenia	71
Clopidogrel	Blood	1997		Hemolytic uremic syndrome*	70
Etanercept	Miscellaneous	1998		Local reactions	198
Infliximab	Gastrointestinal	1998		Increased susceptibility: listeriosis*	158
Meloxicam	CNS-NSAID	2000		Erythema multiforme	107
Montelukast	Respiratory	1998		Churg-Strauss syndrome	220
Orlistat	Miscellaneous	1999		Hypertension	201
Pramipexole	Miscellaneous	1997		Peripheral edema	202
Pramipexole	Miscellaneous	1997		Sleep attacks	207
Quinupristin-Dalfopristin	Antiinfective	1999		Hyponatremia	37
Reboxetine	CNS-antidepressant	2001		Hyponatremia	128
Risedronate	Miscellaneous	1998		Esophageal & gastric ADRs	190
Rivastigmine	Miscellaneous	2000		Pisa syndrome	206

Drug	Drug Class	Year Approve	Interacting Drug	ADR	Page Number
Rofecoxib	CNS-NSAID	1999		Renal failure in transplant patient*	108
Ropinrole	Miscellaneous	1997		Sleep attacks	206, 207
Rosiglitazone	Hormone	1999		Hepatotoxicity	169
Sildenafil	Miscellaneous	1998		Optic neuropathy	208
Sildenafil	Miscellaneous	1998		Priapism in sickle cell*	208
Sirolimus	Miscellaneous	1999		Intersitial pneumonitis	209
Tazarotene (topical)	Skin	1997		Pyogenic granuloma lesion*	232
Thalidomide	Miscellaneous	1998		Toxic epidermal necrolysis*	211, 212
Tolterodine	Miscellaneous	1998	Warfarin	INR prolonged	81
Trastuzumab	Miscellaneous	1998		Serious ADRs	213
Troglitazone	Hormone-diabetics agent	1997		Rheumatoid arthritis exacerbation	169
Troglitazone	Hormone-diabetics agent	1997		Market withdrawal due to ADRs	170
Trovafloxacin	Antiinfective	1999		Neurotoxicity	42
Trovafloxacin	Antiinfective	1999		Eosinophilic hepatitis	43
Trovafloxacin	Antiinfective	1999		Demylinating polyneuropathy*	43
Unoprostone	EENT	2000		Intraocular pressure (increased)	150
Zanamivir	Antiinfective	1999		Respiratory distress	31

* = first report
^ = death

Drug Index

Drug	Drug Class	Class Subset	Page Number
Abacavir	Antiinfective	Antiviral	21
Abciximab	Blood		67
Acetaminophen	CNS	Analgesic-NSAID	101
ADRs	Miscellaneous		187
Alatrovafloxacin	Antiinfective	Quinolone	38
Alendronate	Miscellaneous		190, 191
Allergy immunotherapy	Miscellaneous		191
Allopurinol	Miscellaneous		192
Alosetron	Gastrointestinal		155
Alteplase	Blood		68
Amantadine	Antiinfective	Antiviral	22
Amiodarone	Cardiac		85–87
Amitriptyline	CNS	Antidepressant	122, 123
Amprenavir	Antiinfective	Antiviral	23
Anabolic steroids	Hormone	Steroid	174
Androstenedione	Alternative medicines		3
Anthrax vaccine	Vaccines/serums		235
Antibiotics	Antiinfective	General	17
Antineoplastic	Antineoplastic		51
Antipsychotics	CNS	Antipsychotics	131
Antiretroviral	Antiinfective	Antiviral	20, 21
Antithymocyte globulin	Vaccines/serums		236
Aristolochic acid	Alternative medicines		3
Averrhoa carambola	Alternative medicines		4
Bacitracin	Antiinfective	Miscellaneous	37
Balsalazide	Miscellaneous		193
BCG vaccine	Vaccines/serums		236, 237
Beclomethasone	Respiratory		217
Benzocaine (topical)	Skin		225, 226
Beta-agonists (inhaled)	Respiratory		218
Beta-blockers (ocular)	EENT		147

Drug	Drug Class	Class Subset	Page Number
Doxepin (topical)	Skin		227
Ecabalium elaterium	Alternative medicines		5
Epoetin	Blood		73
Erythomycin	Antiinfective	Macrolide	36
Estrogen	Hormone	Estrogens and miscellaneous	172, 174
Etanercept	Miscellaneous		198
Fenfluramine	Miscellaneous		198
Fentanyl	CNS	Analgesic-opiate	109
Ferrous sulfate	Blood		74
Fluconazole	Antiinfective	Antifungal	18, 19
Fludarabine	Antineoplastic		55
Fluorouracil	Antineoplastic		56
Fluoxetine	CNS	Antidepressant	124
Fluticasone	Respiratory		217, 218
Gabapentin	CNS	Anticonvulsant	114, 115
Gemcitabine	Antineoplastic		56
Gemfibrozil	Cardiac		89
Anesthesia	Miscellaneous		192
Gentamicin	Antiinfective	Aminoglycoside	18
Glimperide	Hormone	Diabetic agent	167
Glyburide	Hormone	Diabetic agent	167
Haloperidol	CNS	Antipsychotic	135, 136
Henna	Alternative medicines		5, 6
Heparin	Blood		74, 75
Hepatitis B vaccine	Vaccines/serums	Vaccine	238, 239
Herbal vitamins	Alternative medicines		6
Ibuprofen	CNS	Analgesic-NSAID	105
Icodextrin	Miscellaneous		199
Imipenem	Antiinfective	Miscellaneous	136
Immune globulin	Vaccines/serums		239, 240
Indinavir	Antiinfective	Antiviral	24, 25
Indomethacin	CNS	Analgesic-NSAID	106
Infliximab	Gastrointestinal		158
Influenza vaccine	Vaccines/serums		241
Interferon-alpha	Antineoplastic		57
Interferon-beta	Antineoplastic		59
Intravenous fluids	Miscellaneous		188, 189
Ipratropium	Respiratory		219
Isotretnoin	Skin		227, 228
Itraconazole	Antiinfective	Antifungal	35
Kampo	Alternative medicines		7
Ketoconazole	Antiinfective	Antifungal	23
Ketoprofen	CNS	Analgesic-NSAID	106
Laminaria tents	Alternative medicines		7

Drug	Drug Class	Class Subset	Page Number
Lamotrigine	CNS	Anticonvulsant	115, 116
Latanoprost	EENT		150
Levofloxacin	Antiinfective	Quinolone	42
Levothyroxine	Hormone	Thyroid	156, 177
Licorice	Miscellaneous		200
Lidocaine	Skin		229, 230
Lithium	CNS	Antipsychotic	136
Ma Huang	Alternative medicines		8
Magnesium sulfate	Miscellaneous		201
Meloxicam	CNS	Analgesic-NSAID	107
Mentholatum	Skin		230
Meperidine	CNS	Analgesic-opiate	110
Metformin	Hormone	Diabetic agent	168
Methadone	CNS	Analgesic-opiate	111
Methotrexate	Antineoplastic		60
Methylprednisolone	Hormone	Steroids	175
Methylsalicylate	Skin		231
Miconazole (vaginal)	Antiinfective	Antifungal	19
Midazolam	CNS	Sedative/hypnotic	140, 141
Milnacipran	CNS	Antidepressant	125
Minocycline	Antiinfective	Tetracycline	46, 47
Misoprostol	Gastrointestinal		159
Mitoxantrone	Antineoplastic		61
Montelukast	Respiratory		220
Morphine	CNS	Analgesic-opiate	111
Nabumetone	CNS	Analgesic-NSAID	107
Naltrexone	CNS	Miscellaneous	143
Nefazodone	CNS	Antidepressant	125
Nifedipine	Cardiac		94
NSAIDs	CNS	Analgesic-NSAID	108
Olanzapine	CNS	Antipsychotic	134, 137
Omeprazole	Gastrointestinal		159, 160
Ondansetron	Gastrointestinal		160
Orlistat	Miscellaneous		201
Oxaliplatin	Antineoplastic		61
Paclitaxel	Antineoplastic		62, 63
Paroxetine	CNS	Antidepressant	126, 127
Pergolide	Miscellaneous		202
Phentermine	Miscellaneous		198
Phenytoin	CNS	Anticonvulsant	117
Phosphate enema	Gastrointestinal		161
Polio vaccine	Vaccines/serums		239
Pramipexole	Miscellaneous		202, 207
Prednisone	Hormone	Steroids	176
Prilocaine	Skin		231
Prochlorperazine	Gastrointestinal		162
Propranolol	Cardiac		95
Propofol	Miscellaneous		203, 204

Drug	Drug Class	Class Subset	Page Number
Propylthiouracil	Hormone	Thyroid	178
Protease inhibitors	Antiinfective	Antiviral	26, 27
Proton pump inhibitors	Gastrointestinal		162
Pseudoephedrine	EENT		148, 151
Psyllium	Gasrtointestinal		163
Quinapril	Cardiac		95
Quinine	Miscellaneous		204
Quinupristin-dalfopristin	Antiinfective	Miscellaneous	37
Ranitidine	Gastrointestinal		163
Reboxetine	CNS	Antidepressant	128
Riluzole	Miscellaneous		205
Rimantadine	Antiinfective	Antiviral	22
Risedronate	Miscellaneous		190
Risperidone	CNS	Antipsychotic	127, 137, 138
Ritonavir	Antiinfective	Antiviral	27–29
Rivastigmine	Miscellaneous		206
Rofecoxib	CNS	Analgesic-NSAID	108
Ropinirole	Miscellaneous		206, 207
Rosiglitazone	Hormone	Diabetic agent	169
Salicylic acid	Skin		232
Saquinavir	Antiinfective	Antiviral	29
Sertraline	CNS	Antidepressant	126
Sildenafil	Miscellaneous		208
Simvastatin	Cardiac		92
Sirolimus	Miscellaneous		209
Sodium polysterene sulfate	Miscellaneous		209
SSRIs	CNS	Antidepressant	128
St. John's wort	Alternative medicines		9–11
Streptokinase	Blood		75
Sulfasalazine	Gastrointestinal		164
Sumatriptan	Miscellaneous		210
Tacrolimus	Miscellaneous		211
Tamoxifen	Antineoplastic		64
Tazarotene (topical)	Skin		232
Temoporfin	Miscellaneous		211
Tetracycline	Antiinfective	Tetracycline	47
Thalidomide	Miscellaneous		211, 212
Theophylline	Respiratory		220
Thioridazine	CNS	Antipsychotic	139
Thyroxine	Hormone	Thyroid	178
Ticlodipine	Blood		75
Timolol	EENT		151
Tolterodine	Miscellaneous		81
Trastuzumab	Miscellaneous		213
Trazodone	CNS	Antidepressant	125
Triamcinolone	Hormone	Steroids	177

Drug	Drug Class	Class Subset	Page Number
Trifluoperazine	CNS	Antipsychotic	129
Trimethoprim-sulfamethoxazole	Antiinfective	Sulfonamide	44
Troglitazone	Hormone	Diabetic Agent	169, 170
Trovafloxacin	Antiinfective	Quinolone	42, 43
Unoprostone	EENT		150
Valacyclovir	Antiinfective	Anti viral	30
Valproate	CNS	Anticonvulsant	117, 118
Valproic acid	CNS	Anticonvulsant	119, 120
Vancomycin	Antiinfective	Miscellaneous	33
Venlafaxine	CNS	Antidepressant	129, 130
Vigabatrin	CNS	Anticonvulsant	121
Vitamins/minerals	Vitamin		183
Warfarin	Blood	Anticoagulant	76–81
Zafirlukast	Respiratory		221
Zanamivir	Antiinfective	Antiviral	31
Zinc	Vitamin		184
Zolpidem	CNS	Sedative/hypnotic	142
Zuclopenthixol	Miscellaneous		213